MERCURY AS A GLOBAL POLLUTANT: HUMAN HEALTH ISSUES

MERCURY AS A GLOBAL POLLUTANT: HUMAN HEALTH ISSUES

Fourth International Conference, August 4–8 1996,
Hamburg, Germany

Edited by

BRIAN WHEATLEY
RON WYZGA

with the editorial assistance of

Billy M. McCormac
Editor-in-Chief

Reprinted from *Water, Air, and Soil Pollution*
Volume 97, Nos. 1–2, June 1997

SPRINGER SCIENCE+BUSINESS MEDIA, B.V.

A C.I.P. Catalogue record for this book is available from the Library of Congress.

ISBN 978-94-010-5760-8 ISBN 978-94-011-3975-5 (eBook)
DOI 10.1007/978-94-011-3975-5

Printed on acid-free paper

Originally published by Kluwer Academic Publishers in 1997
Softcover reprint of the hardcover 1st edition 1997

WATER, AIR AND SOIL POLLUTION / *Volume 97 Nos. 1–2 June 1997*

PART 5
OCCUPATIONAL EXPOSURE

PREFACE

This issue is comprised of papers which were initially presented as part of the Human Health Effects of Methylmercury section at the 4th International Conference on Mercury as a Global Pollutant held in Hamburg, Germany, August 4-8, 1996. The international concern for the human health effects of methylmercury, especially potential effects on the fetus, continues and is the basis for a number of the papers presented in this issue. The papers cover a wide range of topics. Many focus on populations potentially at risk, such as native peoples in Canada, Amazonia and the Seychelles. Others examine industrial exposure in Amazonia and Eastern Europe. Another paper considers the indirect social and cultural impacts of mercury on native peoples in Canada, which is a growing area of concern. Several papers also address the difficult topics of risk assessment and risk management especially with reference to native peoples.

Although in some areas levels of methylmercury in native peoples potentially at risk are falling (parts of Canada), in others, such as Amazonia, they remain elevated. Additionally, as was brought out a number of times during the conference, socio-cultural issues need to be addressed. Indigenous people who rely heavily on natural resources for subsistence are more likely to have their lifestyles disrupted by mercury pollution. This has happened in Canadian Aboriginal communities and appears to be happening in other areas such as the Amazon. Research endeavours must take into consideration the social and cultural repercussions and not simply concentrate on direct health effects known to be associated with high exposure to mercury. These socio-cultural effects are largely qualitative and are less easy to measure. They are influenced by a number of factors including the holistic philosophies and world views held by different cultural groups, perceptions of risk, and communication of information. These factors influence what individuals believe to be the danger or threat and the action taken to reduce the danger. Thus, concern about mercury in food sources may lead to changes in diet from high protein to carbohydrate. Associated with this change in diet are changes in lifestyle, from integrative social activities to more sedentary and less social ones which subsequently contribute to social disruption (violence, substance abuse, suicide). These potential social and cultural impacts of exposure to mercury must be taken into consideration by policy makers and others concerned with setting risk levels which may lead to formal guidelines.

In the area of scientific assessment of risk, there continues to be animated debate on risk assessment and risk management because of the numerous variables involved, the wide range of approaches being taken and variable human susceptibility. However, there was unanimity at the conference that the most sensitive exposure point is the fetus. Therefore, protection of women of child bearing age is essential. However, a balance is required between this need to protect the fetus, when there is still no agreement on effect levels and risk levels, and the need to avoid disruption of the culture and lifestyle of Indigenous peoples through over reaction. This over reaction can result in far greater indirect health impacts on both mother and child than the, to date, theoretical direct effects of methylmercury at levels currently being seen in most parts of the world.

We hope that this special issue will contribute to the ongoing international discussion of these important issues.

Guest Editors

Brian Wheatley

Ron Wyzga

ACKNOWLEDGEMENTS

Our gratitude is extended to the authors who prepared papers for this volume. Equally, our sincerest appreciation is extended to the reviewers for their work and rapid response. All conference participants are indebted to the assistance provided by the sponsors: the Aluminium Company of America (ALCOA); BSL Olefinverbund GMBH; the City of Hamburg; Deutsche Forschungsgemeinschaft; Electric Power Research Institute; Environment Canada: AES; European Commission, SM&T; Florida Department of Environmental Protection; Frontier Geosciences, USA; GKSS Research Centre; Health Canada, MSB; Oak Ridge National Laboratory; US Department of Energy; US Environmental Protection Agency; and Verein der Freunde und Förderer der GKSS. Hundreds of abstracts were evaluated, and organized into a coherent program, by the Conference Technical Advisory Team. For all their efforts we offer our sincerest thanks to the other members of the T.A.T.: Wim Salomons, Willy Baeyens, Nicolas S. Bloom, Alain Boudou, Gustav A. Drasch, Ralf Ebinghaus, William F. Fitzgerald, Cynthia C. Gilmour, Hans Hultberg, Milena Horvat, Åke Iverfeldt, Gerald J. Keeler, Drude Lacerda, Oliver Lindqvist, John Munthe, Gerhard Peterson, Donald B. Porcella, Philippe Quevauviller, John Rudd, William H. Schroeder, Franz Slemr, Ralph Turner, Oleg Vasiliev, Matti Verta and Carl Watras. In large measure, these people were responsible for the quality and success of the conference. We must also express our gratitude to Sylvain Paradis and Jane Boswell-Purdy without whom the process of reviewing papers and assembling this volume, in the time available, would have been next to impossible. The rapid publication of this volume is a tribute to the efforts of the authors, reviewers, and the editorial staff of *Water, Air and Soil Pollution.*

Guest Editors

Brian Wheatley Ron Wyzga

Mercury contamination in hair of riverine populations of Apiacás Reserve in the Brazilian Amazon

Antonio C.Barbosa,[1] Angélica M.Garcia,[2] Jurandir R.de Souza.[1]

[1] Universidade de Brasília, Laboratório de Química Analítica Ambiental, CEP 70919-970, Brasília-DF, Brazil; Phone: 55-61-9846167; Fax: 55-61-2734149; [2] Engevix S/C Ltda.

Abstract. Total and inorganic Hg in 55 samples of hair from riverines, mainly descended from Munduruku and Apiaká Indians, living along the rivers Teles Pires and Juruena have been determined. The sampled population represents 18% of the inhabitants of the region and they eat fish 6 or 7 days a week. Cold-vapor AAS and alkaline digestion with $CdCl_2/SnCl_2$ as reducing agent were employed to estimate total Hg in hair samples. A LDC Analytical, Mod. 1255, Mercury monitor was used for Hg determination. The mean value of total Hg was 34.2μg g^{-1}, with an average of 87.2% of organic Hg. Ninety-three per cent of the sampled population present levels of Hg above 10μg g^{-1}, and 18% over 50μg g^{-1}. A relationship between the mean value of Hg and age of the sampled population is presented. All women at child-bearing age present concentrations of Hg above 10μg g^{-1}. Fifty-four per cent of them had levels over 30μg g^{-1}, with a mean of 41.2μg g^{-1}. For the children under ten years of age, 14% show Hg concentration above 50μg g^{-1}. Comparison of these results with those obtained in 10 other Amazon surveys (n=1672) is shown. The results of the concentration of mercury in fish, mainly piscivorous (n=967) from Amazonian and Wetland (pantanal matogrossense) are also presented, with a mean of 726 ng mg^{-1}. There appears to be a relationship between level of Hg in human and their food ingestion habits.

1. Introduction

About 2,000 ton of the Hg utilized in gold mining sites in the Amazon region during the past 20 years, have been subjected to oxidation and methylation under the favorable conditions found in water and sediments of rivers of that region (Pfeiffer, 1993). As a result of this, the human riverine population has been contaminated with mercury through fish ingestion.

The region has an Indian Reserve with an area of 930,000 hectares and 2,000 inhabitants of the Munduruku tribe. Descendants of the Tupiguarani, which formed the Apiaká tribe, live on the riverbanks of Teles Pires and Juruena. The main diet of this poor and isolated population is fish and manioc. The plantations of corn, manioc and bean being just for subsistence. Hunting wild animals as a protein source, does not take place very often. In addition to Indians and their descendants, that is Munduruku from Pará and Amazonas and Apiaká from Mato Grosso, the population is also formed by people that who went there to extract natural rubber.

The ore material produced in gold mines, by concentrated gravimetric means, is mixed with metallic mercury inside barrels for amalgamation with Hg and then transferred to pans, wherein the gold is washed. The burning of the Hg:Au amalgam is usually done in the open air, without the use of any protecting gear and the solid:liquid waste from the amalgamation is discharged directly to rivers and drainages.

2. Material studied

Fifty-five samples of hair were collected from children and adults, living in the area of the Reserve and its neighbourhood. This was done by sampling, three or four individuals, when possible, from each one of the fifteen riverine families. Considering a population of approximately 300 people, it represents nearly 18% of the inhabitants of that region shown in the map (Fig.1).

Record forms were utilized and archived showing name, place, dietary habits, job, frequency of fish ingestion and kind of fish.

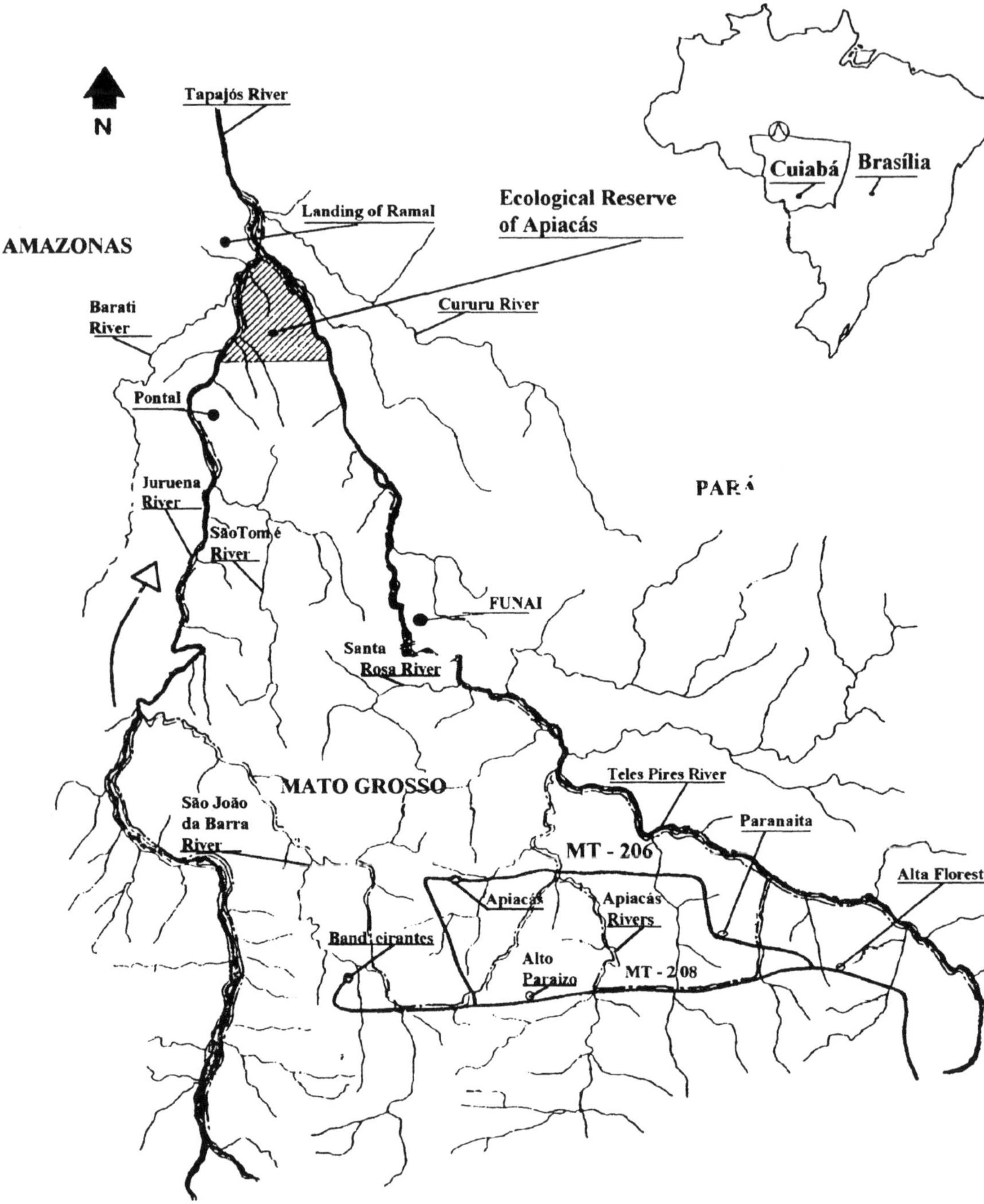

Fig. 1 - Map of the region under survey, showing the sampled Ecological Reserve of Apiacás

3. Method

The procedure utilized in the analysis of total and/or inorganic Hg in hair, was that of Magos and Clarkson, using alkaline digestion (Magos and Clarkson, 1972). The amount of sample taken for Hg analysis was 10-20 mg of hair, weighed into vials previously weighed and labeled. The concentration of Hg was determined by CV-AAS, using a LDC Analytical, Model 1255, Mercury Monitor.

Appraisal of the accuracy of the analytical data was achieved by participating in the Mercury Quality Control Program, Health and Welfare, Ottawa-Canada. Out of the 27 samples analyzed in our laboratory in 1992-1996, 25 (93%) gave results within 2 S.D. and 18 (67%) within 1 S.D. of the corrected mean.

4. Results

Ninety-three per cent of the sampled population present levels of Hg above 10 μg g^{-1} , which is considered as the warning limit, specially for pregnant women (WHO, 1990). The mean value of total Hg was 34.2μg g^{-1} and the median 42.8 μg g^{-1}. The average of organic Hg was 87.2%. The distribution of these results was as follows: 22% between 10 and 20μg g^{-1}, 35% between 20 and 30μg g^{-1}, 18% between 30 and 50μg g^{-1} and finally, 18% over 50μg g^{-1} the level where clinical symptoms may appear (WHO, 1976).

The relationship between the mean value of Hg found and age of the sampled population is shown in Table 1, presenting an increase in the concentration of hair Hg with increasing age.

Table 1

Relationship between the mean of Hg in hair and age of Apiacás population (n = 55)

n	28	21	6
Age (years)	<10	11 - 40	>40
C_{Hg} μg g^{-1} (mean)	29	34	60

All women at child-bearing age (n=13) present concentrations of Hg above 10μg g^{-1} with a mean of 41.2μg g^{-1}. Forty-six per cent of them had levels between 10-30μg g^{-1}, 31% between 30-50 μg g^{-1} and 23% above 50 μg g^{-1}.

For children under ten years old 14% show Hg concentrations above 50μg g^{-1}. Only 14% of them show concentrations below 10μg g^{-1}.

A comparison between the levels of mercury and the sex of the sampled population is shown in Fig. 2. It is worthnoting that the percentage of women is much higher than the percentage of men in the range 30-50 μg g^{-1} of Hg concentration.

Table 2 presents the results of the mercury contamination in hair for the Apiacás region in comparison with the results of the most relevant projects of the Brazilian Amazon region (Barbosa, 1995; Barbosa, 1994; Agaki, 1993; Branches, 1993; Boischio, 1995; Malm, 1994; Agaki, 1995; Forsberg, 1994). The total number of samples was 1672 with a mean value of 34.8μg g^{-1}. If we exclude the results of the Negro River, we obtain a new mean of 15.4 $\mu g\ g^{-1}$ for 1518 hair samples. These results are presented in Fig. 3 and Fig. 4 along with the levels of Hg in fish caught in the same region (mainly piscivorous) (Barbosa, 1995; Boischio, 1995; Malm, 1994; Agaki, 1995; Forsberg, 1994, Filho, 1991). The mean values for both are also shown. The mean was 726 $ng\ g^{-1}$ for the fishs.

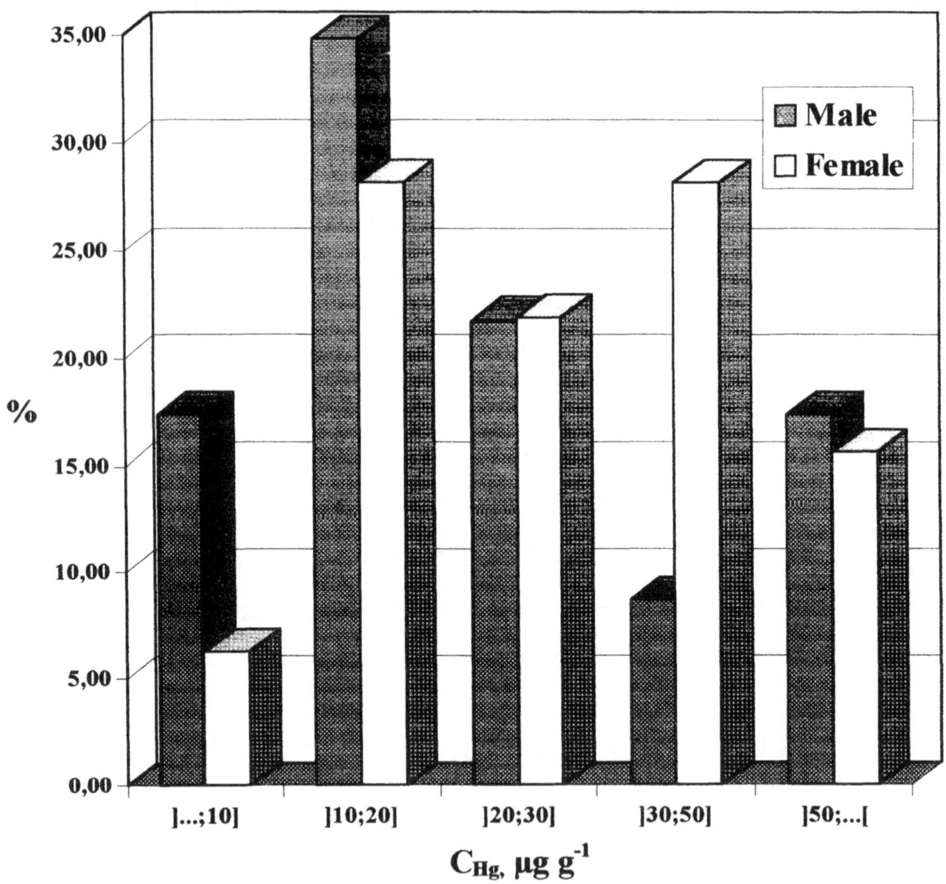

Fig. 2 - Relationship between organic mercury concentration in hair of males (n = 23) and females (n = 32) from Apiacás Reserve.

Table 2

Results of Hg level in hair of riverines from ten surveys in the Amazon Region

Location	n	Mean $\mu g\, g^{-1}$	Maximum $\mu g\, g^{-1}$	Reference
Kayapo Indians	419	8.0	37	Barbosa, 1995; Barbosa, 19944
Cuniã Lake	75	8.7	32	Barbosa, 1995; Boischio, 1995
Tapajós-1/From Rainha to Três Bocas Lake	136	16.3	151	Agaki, 1993
Tapajós-2/Jacareacanga-Ponta de Pedra	114	30.2	151	Branches, 1993
Tapajós-3/River Basin (1986-1994)	256	18.6	176	Malm, 1994
Tapajós-4/Jacareacanga and others villages	51	28.9	52	Agaki,1995
Upper Madeira/Dowstream P. Velho	242	17.2	303	Barbosa, 1995; Boischio, 1995
Madeira/Upstream P. Velho	170	8.9	71	Malm, 1994
Negro/Between Marie and Paduari Rivers	154	75.5	171	Forsberg, 1994
Apiacás/Ecological Reserve	*55*	*34.2*	*128*	
Total	1672	34.8	303	

5. Discussion

The concentration of mercury, in the Amazon rivers, is distinctively higher in the piscivorous species situated at the top of the trophic chain.

The average of total Hg in indians and riverines of the Amazon region, n=1518, whose main diet is fish, was 15.4μg g^{-1}. This figure was obtained excluding, provisionally, the 154 riverines from Negro River that presented levels of Hg extremely high (mean = 75.5 μg g^{-1}), not fully justified as yet if we consider the concentration of Hg found in piscivorous fish of the Negro River (mean = 730 ng g^{-1}) (Forsberg, 1994). Therefore, the mean value found in the hair of riverines of the Ecological Reserve of Apiacás (mean = 34.2 μg g^{-1}), is of concern. Three reasons may explain these high levels. Firstly, the characteristic of the region submitted to heavy mining activities (wherein large uncontrolled amounts of Hg are used to amalgamate gold), mainly from the 80s onward, both upstream (Teles Pires River) and downstream (Tapajós River). Secondly, the strong dependency on fish of the diet of the sampled riverines, ca. 90% claim to ingest fish six times a week. Finally, the commonest ingested fish belongs to the high trophic level, piscivorous, such as Hoplias malabaricus, Serrasalmus spp, Psudoplastystoma fasciatum, Brachyplatystoma spp and Astronotus spp.

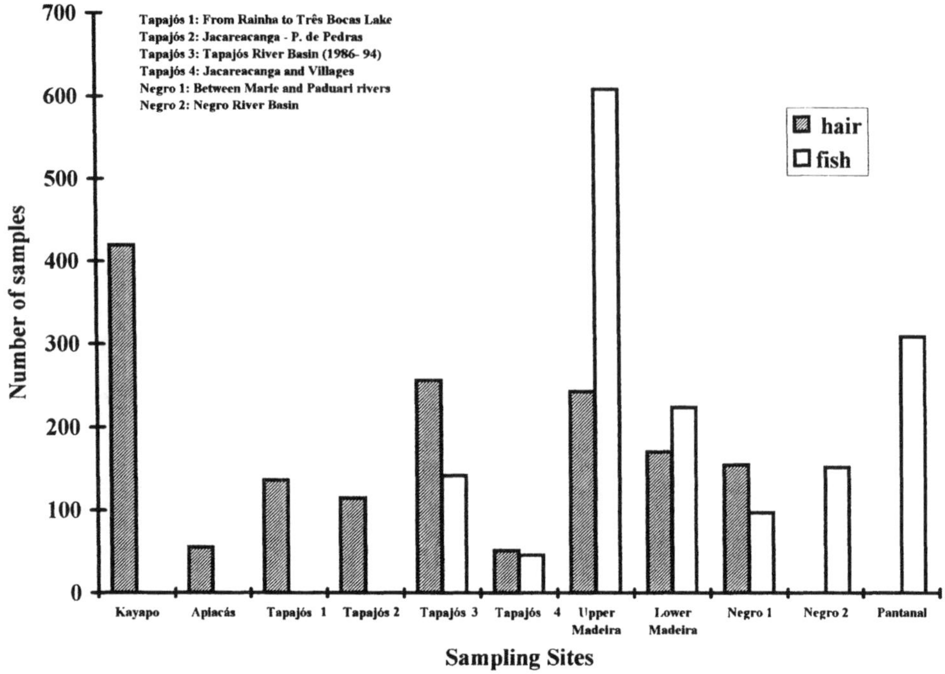

Fig. 3 - Sampling characteristics of hair and fish in various locations of the Amazon Basin

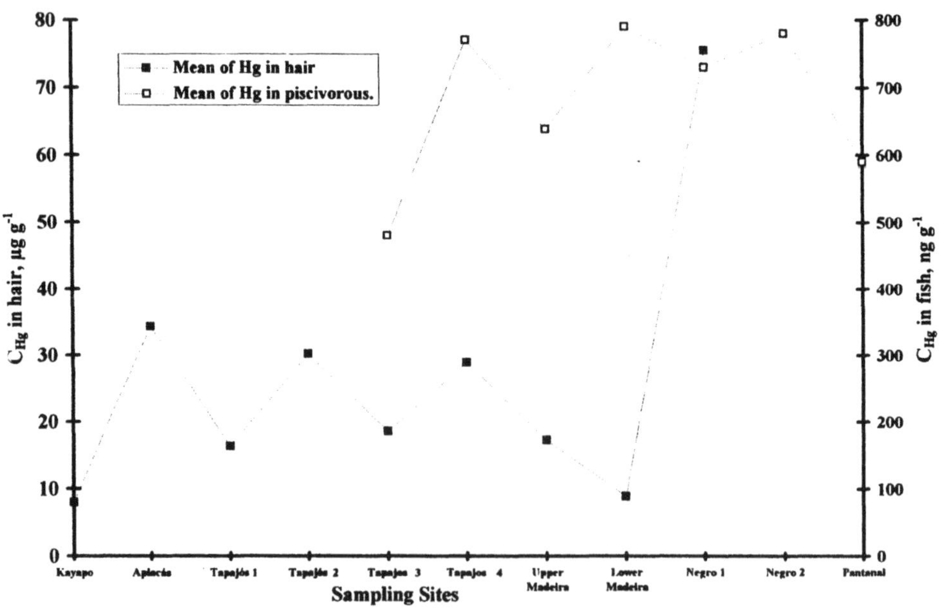

Fig. 4 - Concentrations of Mercury in hair and fish in various locations of the Amazon Basin

6. Recommendations

From the results of this pilot project, some recommendations may be put forward. In the first place, a more comprehensive collection of data is necessary. This can be done by sampling the remaining population. This is being carefully considered in a subsequent expedition, regarding that the Apiacás Reserve is an area difficult of access. On the other hand, the existence of specimens with levels of Hg above 50μg g^{-1} calls for imperative clinical action. In a similar manner, the high Hg levels found in women of child bearing age and in children below 10 years of age, call for urgent medical and social care.

Although the sampled population appears as the more risky group as far as mercurial contamination is concerned, the whole picture of the Amazon region shown in the table 2, is quite serious with ca. 3% of the riverside population presenting levels above 50 μg g^{-1}. The results of 216 samples of fish and 237 of hair from the Madeira river region showed that for 53% of the sampled population, the daily intake of mercury ranged between 0.7 and 3.6 μg kg^{-1}, equivalent to 40-200 μg per person (Boischio, 1995).

Acknowledgments

This research was supported by the Brazilian National Council of Scientific Technological Development (CNPq).

References

Agaki, H., Malm, O., .Branches, F.J.P, Kinjo, Y., Kashima, U., Guimarães, J.R.D., Oliveira, R.B., Haraguchi, K., Pfeiffer, W.C., Takizaswa,U. and Kato, H.: 1995, *Water, Air and Soil Pollution*, **80** 85-94.

Agaki, H., .Malm, O, Kinjo, Y., Harada, M., Branches, F., Pfeiffer, W.C. and Kato, H.: 1993, *Proceedings of the Intern. Symp. on "Assessment of environ. pollution and health effects from methylmercury"*, Nat. Inst. for Minamata Disease, Kumamoto, 41-48.

Barbosa, A.C., Boischio, A.A., East, G.A., Ferrari, I., Gonçalves, A., Silva, P.R.M. and Da Cruz, T.M.E: 1995, *Water, Air and Soil Pollution*, **80**, 109-121.

Barbosa,. A.C., Boischio, A.A., East, G.A., Ferrari I, Gonçalves, A., and Silva, S.R.I.: 1994, *Proceedings of the Intern. Workshop on "Environ. mercury pollution and its health effects in Amazon river basin,* Rio, Env.Agency, Japan, 73-79.

Boischio, A.A., Henshel, D., and Barbosa, A.C.: 1995, *Ecosystem Health*, **1:3**, 177-192.

Branches, F.J.P., .Harada, M, Agaki, H., Malm, O., Pfeiffer, W.C. and Kato, H.: 1993, *Proceedings of the Intern. Symp. on "Assessment of environ. pollution and health effects from methylmercury"*, Nat. Inst. for Minamata Disease, Kumamoto, 19-32

Filho, L.M., Biomagnificação do mercúrio na cadeia trófica, *Ph.D. Thesis*, ERN-UFSCar-Brazil,1991, pp. 208.

Forsberg, B.R., Forsberg, M.C.S., Padovani, C.R., Sargentini, E. and Malm, O.: 1994, *Proceedings of the Intern. Workshop on "Environ. mercury pollution and its health effects in Amazon river basin"*, Rio, Env.Agency, Japan, 33-38.

Magos L. and Clarkson, T.W.: 1972, *J. Assoc. Offic. Anal. Chem.*, **55**, 966-971.

Malm, O., Castro, M.B., .Branches, F.J.P,Zuffo, C.E., Padovani, C., Viana, J.P., Akagi, H., Bastos, W.R., Silveira, E.G., Guimarães, J.D.R. and Pfeiffer, W.C.: 1994, *Proceedings of the Intern. Workshop on "Environmental mercury pollution and its health effects in Amazon river basin*", Rio, Env.Agency, Japan, 25-32.

Pfeiffer, W.C., Lacerda L.D., Salomons W. and Malm O.: 1993, *Environ.Rev.* **1,** 26-37.

WHO: 1976, Environmental Health Criteria I: Mercury, Geneva, *World Health Organization.*

WHO: 1990, Environmental Health Criteria 101 Metthylmercury, Geneva, *World Health Organization.*

Fish contamination and human exposure to mercury in Tartarugalzinho River, Amapa State, Northern Amazon, Brazil. A screening approach

E.D.Bidone[1], Z.C.Castilhos[1], T.J.S. Santos[2], T.M.C. Souza[3] and L.D.Lacerda[1]

[1] Dept. Geoquímica, Universidade Federal Fluminense, Niterói, 24020-007, RJ, Brazil
[2] Curso de Pós-Graduação em Saúde Pública - ENSP - RJ, Brazil
[3] Departamento Nacional da Produção Mineral (DNPM- PA)

Abstract. This study reports for the first time, the Hg concentrations in the fish fauna of the Tartarugalzinho river basin - an important gold mining region in Amapa State, Northern Amazon - and evaluates human exposure to Hg due to fish consumption in the area. We analyzed 16 fish species (carnivorous and omnivorous) common in the aquatic environment of the Tartarugalzinho area and which are mostly consumed by the local population. Mercury concentrations in fish ranged from 35 $\mu g.kg^{-1}$ to 1,225 $\mu g.kg^{-1}$. Among the analyzed fish, 8 species (50%) presented Hg concentrations higher than 500 $\mu g.kg^{-1}$, the U.S. Food and Drug Administration (FDA) Action Level for concentration of Hg in fish. No statistical difference was observed between Hg mean concentrations in carnivorous and omnivorous fish. Within a given species, Hg concentrations were positively correlated with fish size or weight. The Hg concentration ratio between fish and water showed values higher than 50,000. Human exposure was estimated through the daily Hg intake obtained through interviews with the local population on the amount and species of fish consumed and the Hg concentration in the fish. The estimated average daily intake was 114 $\mu g.day^{-1}$. This amount is approximately one-half of the WHO recommended provisional tolerable Hg weekly intake. At screening level, it assumes that there is a level of exposure (e.g, USEPA's RfD = Reference of Dose) below which it is unlikely for even sensitive populations to experience adverse health effects. The estimated exposure level for adult humans (1.6 $\mu g.kg^{-1}.day^{-1}$) was nearly 5 times greater than Hg RfD (0.3 $\mu g.kg^{1}.day^{-1}$). The results suggest a widespread Hg contamination in the local fish fauna. Due to high fish Hg concentrations and high fish intake by local population, environmental exposure to Hg is also high, presenting a health risk to population.

1. Introduction

Gold mining in the Amazon has witnessed intensive migration from traditional sites in southern and western Amazon to new gold fields along the Brazilian-Venezuelan border in recent years. Among these new areas, the Amapa State receives important emissions of Hg from gold mines ("garimpos").

The Tartarugalzinho river basin is located in Amapa State, Brazilian Northern Amazon, approximately at the latitude 00° 00' (Figure 1). 75% of Amapa State is covered by tropical rain forest, 20% by wetlands and flood plain lakes, with low levels of anthropogenic impact. This fact calls for conservation of these very fragile Amazon ecosystems.

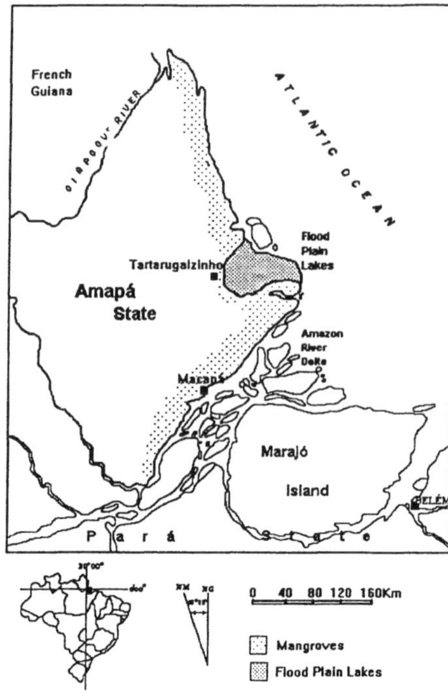

Figure 1. Map of the Study Area.

According to CONEMA-AP (1994): gold mining employs over 15,000 prospectors, ~5% of the Amapa State population. Gold production reaches *c.a.* 1 ton.yr^{-1} and 100% of "garimpos" use Hg, with a Hg/Au relationship in the amalgam higher than 2:1. Therefore, Hg emissions to the local environment can be estimated as between 1 and 2 tons.yr^{-1} (Lacerda & Marins, 1996).

The Tartarugalzinho basin is a key area in this process since: (i) the Tartarugalzinho river flows into flood plain lakes directly linked to mangroves with very high biological productivity; (ii) local human groups still depend on fish as major protein source; (iii) local limnological conditions favor Hg methylation; (iv) the Tartarugalzinho constitutes the most important biological reserve in the Amapa State, due to its unique ecosystem types.

The general population is primarily exposed to MeHg through fish consumption. In this study we report for the first time on the Hg concentrations in the local fish fauna and evaluate potential human exposure to Hg due to fish consumption in the area. This work is a screening, i.e., rapidly identifying potentially important factors or phenomena to enable the elimination of those of lesser significance (IAEA, 1990).

2. Materials and Method

The 45 fish samples considered in this study are representatives of the 16 species (9 carnivorous and 7 omnivorous) caught and commercialized in the study area. Fish samples

were collected from the Tartarugalzinho river and from the Duas Bocas lake (see outline Figure 2).
Each fish was weighed, and its length was measured at the time of collection. The samples were put in polyethylene bags and frozen. Mercury was analyzed in the fish muscle through Atomic Absorption Spectrophotometer technique (A-G/VARIAN MODEL) using the Vapor Generation Acessory-VGA (CVAAS). The samples were digested in sulpho-nitric solution in the presence of vanadium pentoxid 0.1%; the oxidation completed by adding potassium permanganate 6% until the fixation of the violet colour. Immediately before the determination, the excess of permanganate was reduced with hidroxilamine 50% (Campos, 1990). Reference standard IAEA-fish muscle tissue with a certified Hg concentration of 0.74±0.13 $\mu g.g^{-1}$ were also analyzed, giving a value of 0.73±0.08 $\mu g.g^{-1}$ (n=4).
Water and sediments were also collected in the area using clean procedures, and were analyzed through CVAAS. Water samples were analyzed unfiltered, giving the total (dissolved + particulate).

3. Results and Discussion

GOLD MINES ("GARIMPOS") OF TARTARUGALZINHO

Gold deposits of Tartarugalzinho are exploited at the surface and underground near the surface, from alluvial placers material. In order to avoid the direct emission of Hg to the Tartarugalzinho river, a rough tailing dam was constructed in the mining site. However, some effluent can reach the Tartarugalzinho river from a small affluent that crosses the "garimpo" area, the Candido Stream, and from creeks arising from cracks in the dam.
The Tartarugalzinho river flows into the Duas Bocas lake which is part of a flood plain lakes ecosystem.

CONCENTRATION OF HG IN SEDIMENT AND WATER

A preliminary survey on Hg concentrations in sediment and water (Figure 2), showed a Hg concentration gradient in the Candido Stream sediments, with values ranging from 1.6 $mg.kg^{-1}$ up stream of the dam to 0.03 $mg.kg^{-1}$ at the mouth of the stream at the Tartarugalzinho river junction, below the dam. The Hg concentrations in the Tartarugalzinho river sediments were lower than 0.03 $mg.kg^{-1}$, whereas the dam sediments presented Hg values of 10 $mg.kg^{-1}$ (the quantity of Hg stocked in the dam was estimated as about 2.5 tons). This fact favors the positive action of the tailing dam in controlling Hg effluents. The mercury in the sediment is essentially as metallic mercury (Hg^{o}).
Water draining the tailings dam (DW) shows total (dissolved + particulate) Hg concentrations of 2.0 $\mu g.l^{-1}$ and is about 4 times lower than the direct effluent water from "garimpos" reaching the tailing dam (GC=7.5 $\mu g.l^{-1}$). Average Hg concentration in well drinking water (WD) is 1.1$\mu g.l^{-1}$. This value is approximately 5 times higher than the maximum admissible value established for the Brazilian water legislation (0.2$\mu g.l^{-1}$).
Total mercury concentrations in the Tartarugalzinho river water (TR) are affected by suspended solids (SS) concentrations. Concentrations ranging from a maximum of 0.8 Hg $\mu g.l^{-1}$, at stations near the "garimpos", with SS concentrations of 150 $mg.l^{-1}$, to a minimum

of <0.03 Hg µg.l^{-1} at stations with very low SS concentrations (SS<50 mg.l^{-1}). This strongly suggests that most Hg flowing the river is associated with suspended solids.
Total Hg concentrations in water of the Duas Bocas lake also depend on suspended solids concentrations. When SS increased due to ressuspension of lake sediments, the Hg concentration averaged 0.05 µg.l^{-1}. With low SS, Hg concentration change to values lower than 0.03 µg.l^{-1}. This fact suggests a contamination of Duas Bocas lake sediments with Tartarugalzinho river sediments and/or with atmospheric inputs.

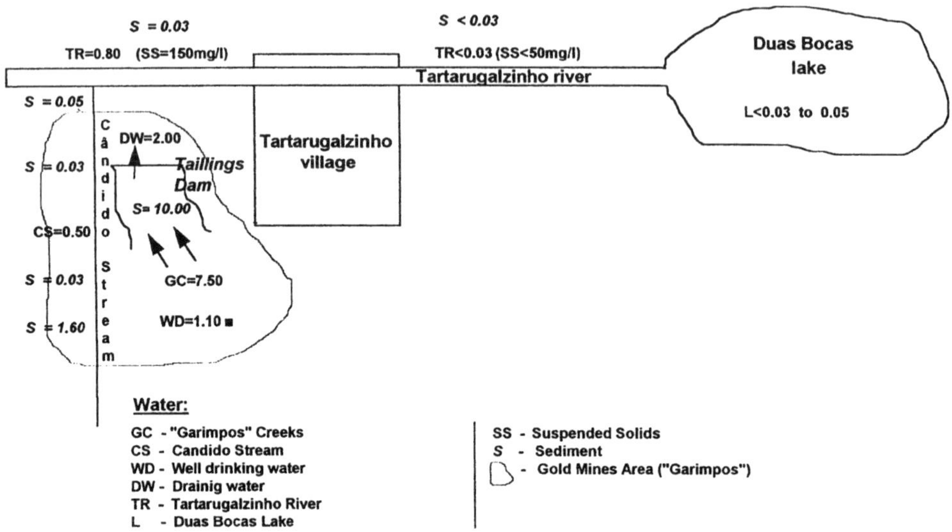

Figure 2 - Mercury concentrations in total water (µg/l) and in sediments (mg/kg)

MERCURY CONCENTRATIONS IN FISH

The fish samples considered in this study are representatives of the 16 main species (9 carnivorous and 7 omnivorous) caught and commercialized in the study area (Table 1).

Table I. Mercury concentrations in fish from the Tartarugalzinho basin.

Common name (n)=number of samples	Scientific name	Hg concentration (μg/Kg)
CARNIVOROUS		
Aruanã (2)	Osteoglossum	329
Ituí (1)	Sternopigus sp.	305
Jacundá (2)	Crenicichla sp.	719
Jeju (1)	Erythrinus erythrinus	541
Piranha (8)	Serrassalmus sp.	742±460
Pirarucu (1)	Arapaima sp.	880
Traíra (2)	Hoplias malabaricus	335
Tucunaré (6)	Cichla sp.	441±200
Ueua (1)	Acestrorhyncus sp.	786
Carnivorous (24)		Mean=605±200
OMNIVOROUS		
Aracu (1)	Laemolyta sp.	35
Cachorro de Padre (1)	Parauchemipterus galeatus L	673
Cará (6)	Cichlasoma sp.	251±202
Mandubé (1)	Ageneiosus sp.	342
Matrinxão (4)	Brycon sp.	263±102
Pacu Branco (6)	Myleus sp.	608±114
Taumatá (2)	Hoplosternum thoracatum	1225
Omnivorous (21)		Mean = 534±376

The mean concentration of Hg in carnivorous species from this work was similar to that from carnivorous species from Amazon contaminated rivers (Lacerda & Solomons, 1991; Lacerda et al., 1994; Malm et. al., 1996). Among the analyzed fish, 8 species (50%) presented Hg concentrations higher than 500 $\mu g.kg^{-1}$, the U.S. Food and Drug Administration (FDA) Action Level for concentration of Hg in fish. Within a given species (eg., *Serrassalmus* sp. and *Cichla* sp.), Hg concentrations were positively correlated with fish weight (nonparametric Spearman correlation test: $p < 0.05$). Moreover, the Hg concentration ratio between fish/water showed values higher than 50,000. These observations strongly suggest that Hg is accumulated as MeHg in the local fish fauna. Moreover it is necessary to consider the lake metabolic processes. Mason et al. (1995) suggested that most of the discrimination between inorganic and MeHg occurs during trophic transfer while the major enrichment factor is between water and phytoplankton. As a result, MeHg concentrations in fish are ultimately determined by water chemistry which controls MeHg speciation and uptake at the base of the food chain. It is generally agreed that Hg concentrations in carnivorous fish are higher than in non-carnivorous species. Surprisingly, no statistical difference was observed between Hg mean levels of carnivorous and omnivorous fish, in this work, although the relatively small number of samples and the non-normalization by size or weight hamper any generalization.

HUMAN EXPOSURE FROM FISH CONSUMPTION

The general population is primarily exposed to MeHg through the diet. Fish and fish products are the dominant source of MeHg in the diet. In the present study the estimated average daily intake is 114 $\mu g.day^{-1}$. This value was obtained by multiplication of mean Hg concentration in fish - 569 $\mu g.kg^{-1}$ in this study - by local adult human ingestion rate of $0.2 kg.day^{-1}$ (SUDEPE, 1988). For purpose of estimating the average daily intake of MeHg from fish, it was assumed that 80% of Hg concentration in fish is MeHg (WHO, 1990). Most previous studies on MeHg in Amazon fish showed that it frequently represents from 70% to 95% of the total Hg content of fish (Akagi et al., 1994). Thus, the estimated average daily intake for MeHg in this study is approximately 100 $\mu g.day^{-1}$. This amount is one-half of the recommended provisional tolerable mercury weekly intake (200 $\mu g.day^{-1}$ WHO, 1989).
According to WHO (1990), the steady-state Hg concentration in blood (C) in $\mu g.l^{-1}$ is related to the average daily dietary intake (d) in µg Hg, as follows: $C = 0.95 * d$.
Hair concentrations of MeHg are proportional to blood concentrations at the time of formation of the hair strand. In general, the concentration in hair is 250 times the simultaneous concentration in blood. It should be emphasized that single-compartment model refers to the "average" adult human with a body weight of 70 kg. Clearly this model is only an approximation to the more complex kinetics of Hg distribution and metabolism, a process which is known to follow multiphasic kinetics (Berlin, 1986). A blood MeHg level about 200 $\mu g.l^{-1}$, corresponding to 50 $\mu g.g^{-1}$ of hair, has been associated with a low risk (5%) of neurological damage to adults and no adverse effects have been detected with long-term daily MeHg intakes of 3-7 $\mu g.kg^{-1}$ body weight (WHO, 1990).
In this study, taking into account an adult human population and their estimated average daily Hg intake (114 $\mu g.day^{-1}$), the blood Hg levels estimated and hair Hg levels estimated are about 108 $\mu g.l^{-1}$ and 27 $\mu g.g^{-1}$, respectively. This estimate agrees with the results reported by Akagi et al. (1994) on hair Hg levels in the Tartarugalzinho population. These authors reported total Hg and MeHg in hair samples of the local humans ranging between 8.4 and 53.8 $\mu g.g^{-1}$, with a mean value of 28±13.3 $\mu g.g^{1}$. The predominant form of hair Hg was MeHg (92%). However, a pregnant women may suffer effects at lower MeHg exposure levels than no pregnant adults, suggesting a greater risk for pregnant women. WHO (1990) recommends epidemiological studies on children exposed in utero to levels of MeHg that result in peak maternal hair Hg levels below 20 $\mu g.g^{-1}$, in order to screen for those effects only detectable by available psychological and behavioral tests.
Moreover, at screening level, a Hazard Quotient (HQ) approach developed based on EPA's (1989) Risk Assessment Guidance For Superfund assumes that there is a level of exposure (i.e. RfD) below which it is unlikely for even sensitive populations to experience adverse

health effects. HQ is defined as the ratio of a single substance exposure level (E) to a reference dose (E/RfD). When HQ exceeds unity, there may be concern for potential health effects. In the present study, the estimate exposure level for adult humans (1.6 $\mu g.kg^{-1}.day^{-1}$) is about 5 times greater than Hg RfD:0.3$\mu g.kg^{-1}.day^{1}$ (IRIS, 1993).
The results suggest widespread Hg contamination in the local fish fauna. Due to high fish Hg concentrations and high fish intake by local population, environmental exposure to Hg is also high, presenting a health risk to this population.

References

Akagi, H., Yoshihide, K., Branches, F., Malm, O., Harada, M., Pfeiffer, W.C., and Kato, H.: 1994, Methylmercury Pollution in Tapajos River Basin, Amazon, Environmental Sciences (3): 25-32

Berlin, M.: 1986, Mercury. In: Friberg, L., Nordberg, G.F. and Voulk, V., ed. Handbook on the toxicology of metals, 2nd ed.; Elsevier Science Publishers, pp. 387-445.

Campos, R.C. and Curtis, A.J.: 1990. In: Riscos e Consequências do Uso de Mercúrio, Seminário Nacional, FINEP, Rio de Janeiro, pp. 110-134.

CONEMA- Coordenadoria Estadual do Meio Ambiente do Estado do Amapá: 1994, Diagnóstico do Setor Ambiental do Estado do Amapá, 28p.

EPA- Environmental Protection Agency: 1989, Risk Assessment Guidence For Superfund.vol 1. chapt.7, pp. 1-20.

IAEA- International Atomic Energy Agency: 1990, Safety Series, nº 100, 105p.

IRIS- Integrated Risk Information System: 1993, EPA, Office of Research and Development, Washington, DC.

Lacerda, L.D. and Solomons, W.:1991, Dutch Ministry of Housing, Physical Planning and Environment, Chemical Time Bomb Project.

Lacerda, L.D., Bidone, E.D, Guimarães, A.F. and Pfeiffer, W.C..: 1994, Anais da Academia Brasileira de Ciências. **3** (66).374-379.

Lacerda, L.D. and Marins, R.V.: 1996, J. Geochem. Explor. (in press).

Malm, O., Guimarães, J.R.D., Castro, M.B., Bastos, W.R., Viana, J.P., Branches, F.J.P., Silveira, E.G. and Pfeiffer, W.C.: 1996, Fourth International Conference on Mercury as a Global Pollutant, Hamburg, Germany, August 4-8, Abstract p.10.

Mason, R.P., Reinfelder, J.R. and Morel, F.M.M.: 1995, Water, Air and Soil Pollution, **80**:915-921.

SUDEPE: 1988, Diagnostico do setor pesqueiro. 81p.

WHO: 1989, Evaluation of certain food additives and contaminants. Thirty-third report of the Joint FAO/WHO Expert Committee on Food Additives, Geneva, World Health Organization (WHO Technical Report Series 776).

WHO:1990, Environmental Health Criteria 101: Methylmercury. Geneva, World Health Organization

Methylmercury in hair samples from different riverine groups, Amazon, Brazil

Kehrig. H.A., Malm, O. and Akagi, H.*

Laboratório de Radioisótopos Eduardo Penna Franca, Instituto de Biofísica Carlos Chagas Filho, Centro de Ciências da Saúde, UFRJ, 21941 - 900 Rio de Janeiro
**Department of Epidemiology, National Institute for Minamata Disease (NIMD) 4058 - 18, Hama. Minamata, Kumamoto 867 Japan*

Abstract:

The present study was aimed to evaluate comparatively the levels of methylmercury (MeHg) in human hair, collected from different groups of Amazonian populations exposed to contamined fish. The study was undertaken in fishing villages and gold mining areas, mainly in the Tapajós and Madeira river basins, two of the main tributaries of Amazon river. The study population included 125 hair samples, chosen from a collection of over one thousand samples collected in different periods. Hair analyses were conducted with a new efficient extraction technique and measured with ECD-gas chromatographer. This analytical method presented good accuracy and precision when compared with standard hair samples from IAEA. A highly significant correlation was found at the interlaboratory exercise between National Institute for Minamata Disease and our laboratory at Federal University of Rio de Janeiro. The results of the present study showed, through hair analysis, a relationship between environmental contamination by mercury and methylmercury and dietary habits of the Amazon population. The highest levels of MeHg in hair samples were found in riverine population from upper Tapajós river and in riverine population from some tributaries of Madeira river, followed by population of fishing villages from Madeira river. Majority of the women of child-bearing age presented high MeHg concentration in hair samples (10 $mg.kg^{-1}$). On the other hand, Yanomami Indians presented MeHg concentration below the limit tolerable of 6 $mg.kg^{-1}$.

1. Introduction

Mercury (Hg) released by gold mining is polluting several ecosystems of river basins in Brazilian Amazon. Environmental mercury pollution due to gold mining, locally known as *garimpos,* comes from the use of enormous amount of metallic mercury (Hg^0) to amalgamate the fine gold particles. This mercury is being discharged in aquatic systems during gold prospecting and also to the atmosphere, in this case exposing people to mercury vapour. Mercury released to the atmosphere after burning of amalgam undergoes oxidation and partly return to the aquatic environment by wet and dry precipitation (Lindqvist *et al.*, 1984).

Though, inorganic mercury, Hg^{+2}, is converted to methylmercury (MeHg), the most toxic mercury compound, by bacteria in sediment (Guimarães *et al.*, 1995), and is then bioaccumulated in fish and biomagnified up through the aquatic food chain and to the humans at one top end (Malm *et al.*, 1990, WHO, 1990).

The major source of human exposure to methylmercury is through the consumption of fish and fish products (WHO, 1990).In the Amazon region, the riverine communities depend heavily on fish as the main component of their diet and are not exposed to inorganic mercury vapour. In Brazil, for the general population, daily Hg intake through fish consumption ranged from 5 to 100 $\mu g.kg^{-1}$ body weight with a median of 30 $\mu g.kg^{-1}$ body weight, with exposure times lasting from several months to years (Boischio, A.A. *et al.*, 1995).

One of the main target organ for MeHg is the central nervous system (CNS) for both adults and foetus (Tsubaki & Takahashi, 1986). The developing brain is much more vulnerable and sensitive to the effects of methylmercury (Choi, 1989). Clinical symptoms of MeHg poisoning in children and adults include paresthesias, ataxia, dysarthria, impairment of hearing, tremor in the limbs and constriction of visual field (Tsubaki & Takahashi, 1986, WHO, 1990). MeHg level of 50 to 125 $mg.kg^{-1}$, in hair, is considered the minimum level at which clinical symptoms may occur (WHO,1976)

Scalp hair is a useful bioindicator of methylmercury exposure (Cammer *et al.*, 1979). Because MeHg is incorporated into the forming hair, and correlates with the MeHg concentration in blood. Thus the concentration profile along the hair strand represents a recapitulation of previous blood concentrations, i.e. previous MeHg exposure (WHO, 1990)

People living near gold mining areas and depending on the local fish as a protein source may be exposed to both inorganic and methylmercury. Therefore in order to better understand the methylmercury cycle, a reliable and simple methodology was developed by Akagi and Nishimura (1991) and implanted in Brazil.

Therefore, the present study was aimed to use a new simple and efficient extraction technique developed for methylmercury analysis in hair samples. Furthermore, the another aim of this study was to evaluate more precisely the levels of MeHg in human hair collected from different groups of people living in fishing villages and gold mining areas mainly in the Tapajós and the Madeira river basins, two of the main tributaries in the Amazon river system.

2. Material and Methods

During the last 10 years the UFRJ laboratory had been working in several different areas in the Amazon and collected a big number of samples. From this hair samples collection we choose more representative groups of individuals, based on previous total Hg data, better information on alimentary habits and no other Hg exposure source.

A total of 125 human hair samples were selected from a collection of over one thousand samples collected, in different periods, from different groups of people living in fishing villages and gold mining areas along the Tapajós river basin (Jacareacanga and Brasília Legal), and the Madeira river basin (Humaitá and Manicoré), from riverine population of two tributaries of the Madeira river and from Yanomami Indians from Roraima state.

These areas (Figure 1), in Brazilian Amazon region, present different levels of mercury inputs from gold mining areas.

2.1. Analytical methodology

Analytical procedures described here were developed at the National Institute for Minamata Disease (NIMD) and adapted at Federal University of Rio de Janeiro (UFRJ).

Methylmercury in hair was extracted with 2 N hydrochloric acid (5 ml at 100°C for 5 minutes) in extremely fine cut hair (10 to 20 mg) wetted with 2 drops of ethanol (to break surface tension). After cooling at temperature room, 1 ml of this acid extract was transferred to a 10 ml test tube and MeHg was extracted with 4 ml of benzene during 5 minutes. The benzene extract was measured with ECD - gas chromatographer under the following conditions: glass packed column with support Hg-20 (UNIPORT HP - Japan) used with oven temperature at 150°C, injection port temperature at 180°C and detector at 200°C. Nitrogen (carrier gas) flow rate in the column was 40 ml/min (Akagi & Nishimura, 1991).

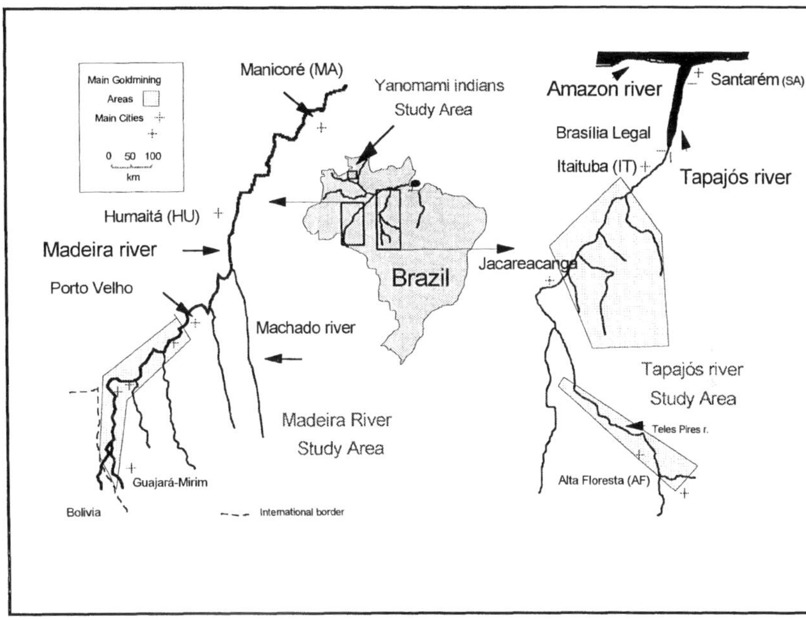

Figure 1. Study Area

3. RESULTS

3.1 Intercalibration exercises

Results of the analysis performed at the National Institute for Minamata Disease (NIMD) and at our laboratory at Federal University of Rio de Janeiro (UFRJ) are presented in Figure 2, for hair samples collected at Jacareacanga (Tapajós river basin). Comparison between the two laboratories showed good agreement with highly significant correlation ($r^2 = 0.9786$), and the paired "t" test showed they are similar, in which $t_{0.05(2),27} = 2.052$ and $0.25 < P(t_{27} \leq 1.501) < 0.10$.

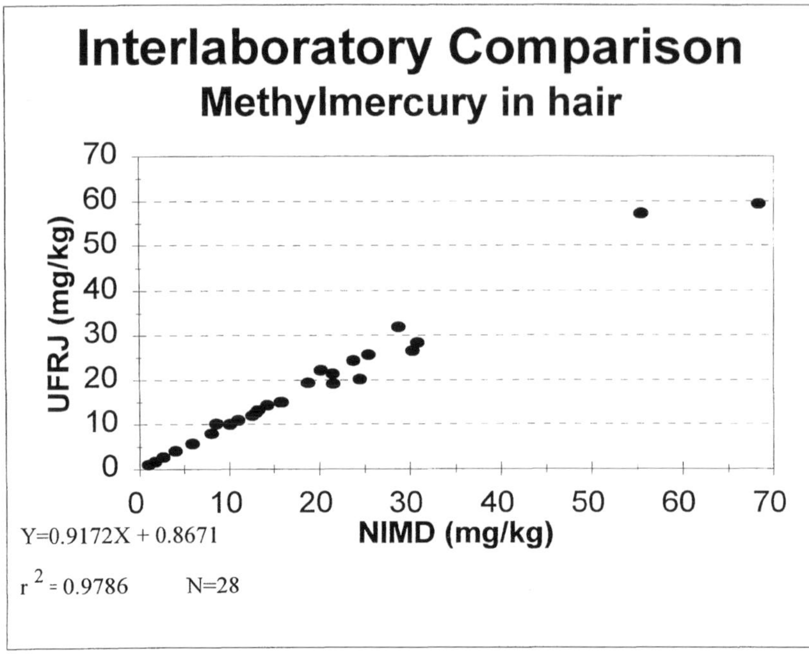

Figure 2:Correlation of MeHg analysis between NIMD and UFRJ

Precision and accuracy of the analytical method were demonstrated with a comparison exercise with two standard samples from International Atomic Energy Agency (IAEA). The results of analysis of certified standard samples are shown in Table I.

Table I: MeHg Concentration in certified standard hair sample (mg.kg^{-1}):

Sample	Certified value mean ± SD range	UFRJ value mean ± SD range
IAEA 085 sample 486	21.60 ± 4.20 (20.10 - 23.00)	20.50 ± 1.91 (18.10 - 23.60)
IAEA 086 sample 376	0.291 ± 0.092 (0.254 - 0.329)	0.308 ± 0.038 (0.245 - 0.36)

As far as we know this is the first time certified direct methylmercury analysis done on a routine basis in Brazil.

3.2 Hair sample

The results of the levels and percentages of methylmercury in hair population groups from different river basins, are summarised in Table II, with the average values, but also the range of values. All these population groups have fish as their main protein source. The average weekly consumption of fish range from 4 to 7 times per week.

TableII: MeHg Concentration in hair from Brazilian Amazon populations.

Sampling Point	Date	N	MeHg (mg.kg^{-1} d.w.) average ± SD	(min. - max.)	% MeHg average	(min. - max.)
Jacareacanga	1992	30	17.63 ± 13.64	(1.00 - 59.40)	88.1	(32.0 - 100.0)
Brasília Legal	1994	25	16.54 ± 7.19	(8.29 - 33.38)	82.7	(68.3 - 100.0)
Humaitá	1990	11	9.18 ± 5.00	(4.27 - 21.51	70.6	(34.0 - 89.4)
	1991	12	6.14 ±1.74	(2.78 - 8.85)	56.6	(28.7 - 75.2)
Manicoré	1990	10	10.88 ± 5.73	(5.30 - 23.21)	75.2	(8.7 - 97.0)
	1992	10	11.49 ± 3.82	(6.45 - 19.70)	69.5	(57.4 - 83.9)
Riverine people from Madeira river tributaries	1994	7	21.79 ± 14.14	(4.63 - 41.76)	84.9	(68.4 - 96.9)
	1995	6	28.59 ± 6.63	(17.47 - 37.84)	61.1	(39.2 - 73.2)
Yanomami	1990	14	3.32 ± 1.23	(1.51 - 5.99)	77.3	(59.7 - 97.2)

In the Tapajós river basin, the estimated average daily consumption of fish, per capita (adults), was around 160 grams (David Cleary, *personnal communication*). And in Madeira river basin, Boischio *et al.* (1995) estimated the daily fish consumption, per capita, throughout the year to be around 200 grams per day. Thus the current estimate of MeHg intake can be compared with Hg concentrations found in fish and hair samples (Clarkson, 1988).

The MeHg analysis for hair samples from Jacareacanga and Brasília Legal, in the upper Tapajós river showed high average values, around 17.00 mg.kg^{-1} and the average percentages of MeHg to total Hg were more than 80%, indicating that organic mercury was the predominant form of mercury that people were exposed through the consumption of contaminated fish with methylmercury.

Figure 3 presents the average of methylmercury levels in child and adults from Jacareacanga and Brasília Legal. Both child and adults male averages, from Jacareacanga and Brasília Legal, are higher than the female averages.

Adults generally consumed fish more frequently than children and males tended to consume this organism more often than females.

The results presented in these populations living on Tapajós river are similar to the ones reported previously in Akagi *et al.* (1994) and Lebel *et al.* (1996), particularly concerning the MeHg percentages and MeHg averages. Similar slight differences between men and women have been reported (Airey, 1983; Lebel *et al.*, 1996).

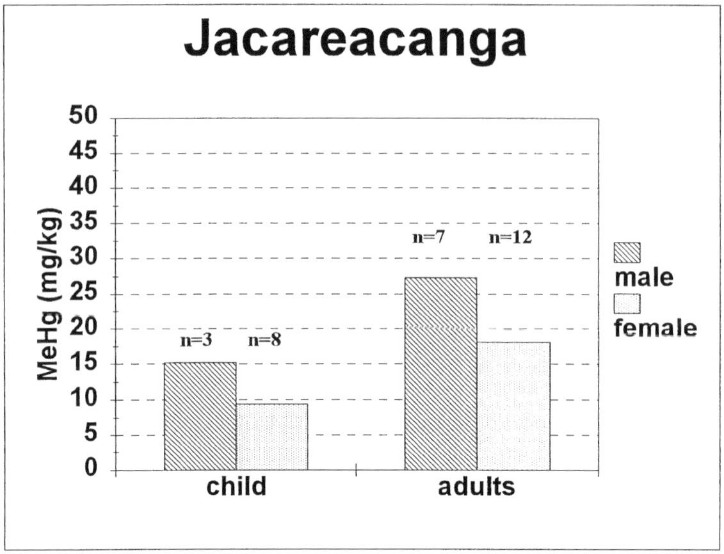

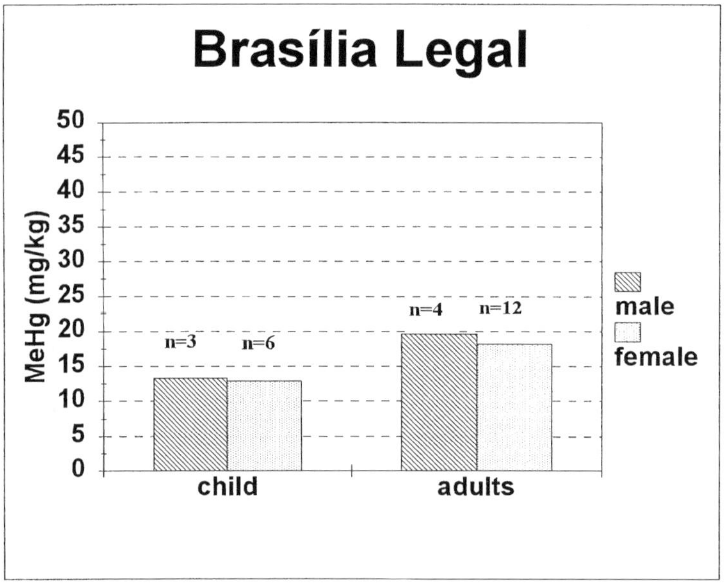

Figure 3: Methylmercury concentration, mean and standard deviation in human hair from Tapajós river basin

Figure 4 shows the frequency distribution of methylmercury concentration ranges in women of child - bearing age (14 - 45 years old) from the same two fishing villages in the upper Tapajós river. More than 75% of these females presented methylmercury levels ranging from 10 and 30 $mg.kg^{-1}$ in their hairs. Maternal exposure at a range between 10 and 20 $mg.kg^{-1}$ as measured by maternal hair concentration increase risk to the foetus, around of 5% risk (Cox *et al.*, 1989, WHO,1990, Girard and Dumont, 1995).

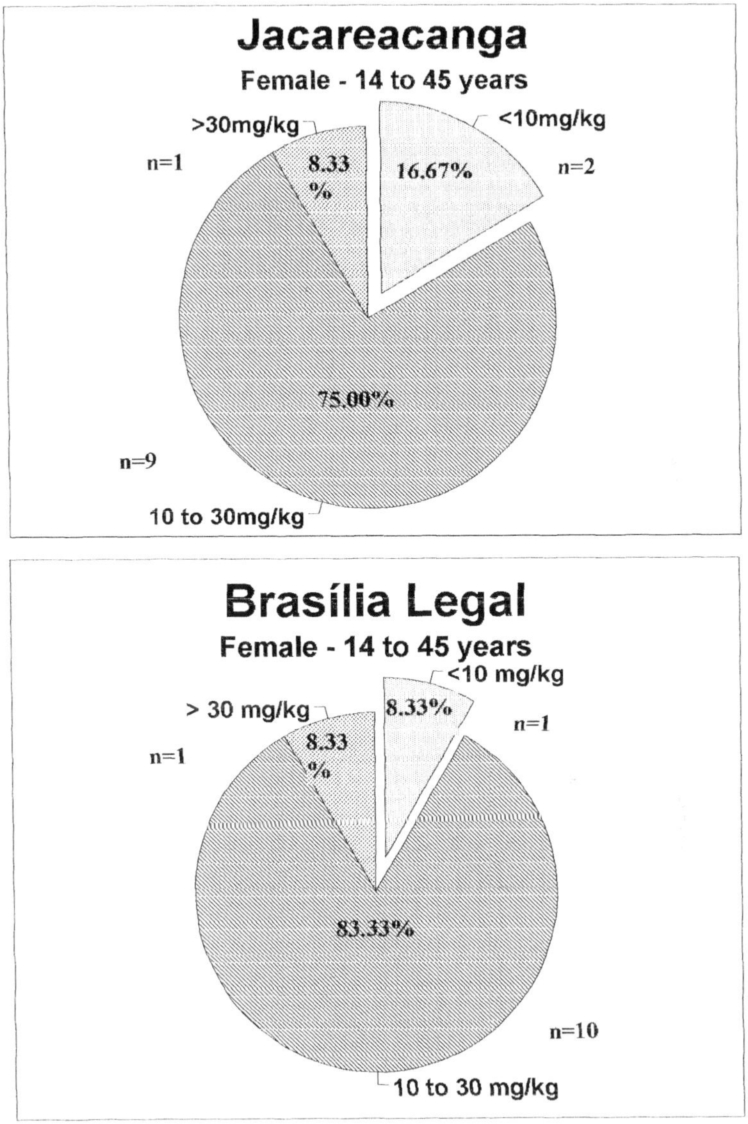

Figure 4: Distribution of methylmercury in human hair from Tapajós river basin

In populations that consume large amounts of fish, more than 100g per day, the hair levels of MeHg in women of child - bearing age should be monitored (WHO, 1990).

The longitudinal analysis of mercury and methylmercury along hair strands provides information on previous methylmercury exposure in individual (WHO,1990). Since hair grows about 1.0 to 1.5 cm per month, past information on Hg exposure is possible over several months or years depending the length of hair sample (Akagi *et al.*, 1994; Akagi *et al.*, 1995a).

Figure 5 shows the results of such a longitudinal analysis of hair methylmercury in a group of female with different ages from Brasília Legal. In this study, we consider that hair grows about 1.0 cm per month.

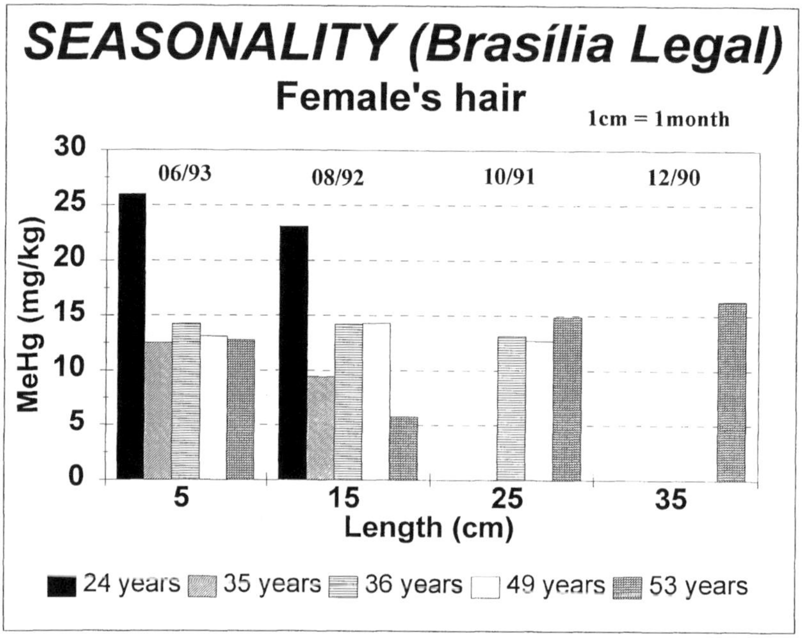

Figure 5 : Longitudinal MeHg analysis along hair strands collected in November 1994

Figure 6 presents the results of a longitudinal analysis of hair total mercury and methylmercury in a young women with 14 years old from Brasília legal.

In a general way in the Amazon region, May to October is the dry season, and the rainy season lasts for the remaining half of the year. Considering these results individuals were exposed continuously to methylmercury at fairly constant levels at least in the last few years up to the time of sampling with some seasonal variations.

The populations, from the upper Tapajós river, have a higher ingestion of big carnivorous fish at the end rainy season (Malm *et al.*, 1995).

Seasonal variations in hair levels were also observed confirming previous studies (Akagi *et al.* 1995b; Lebel *et al.* 1996).

By the analyses of human hair, Akagi *et al.* (1995b) found a seasonal and temporal change in MeHg concentration. The concentration is higher in dry season and it was thought to be either because higher intake of fish, higher mercury concentration in fish, or more intense gold mining activity in dry season.

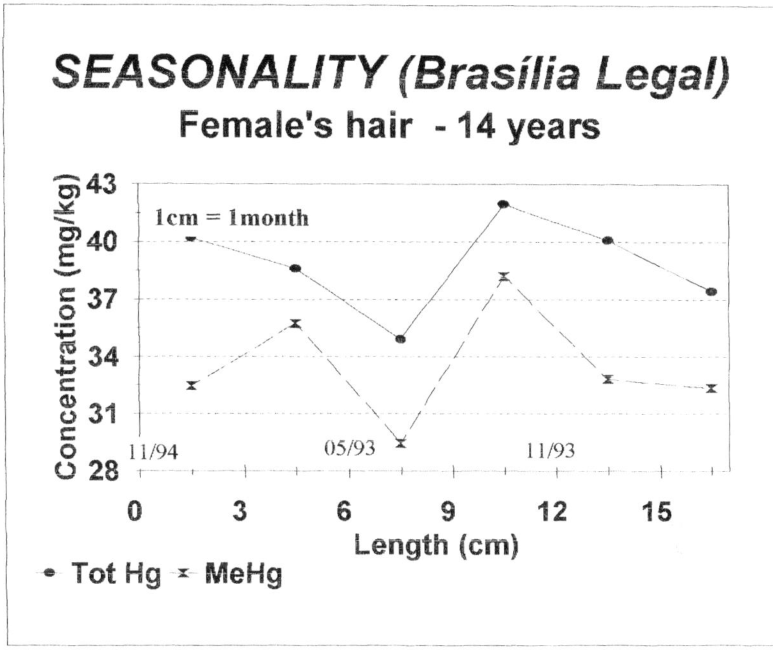

Figure 6: Longitudinal MeHg analysis along hair strands collected in November 1994

Figure 7 presents the distribution of methylmercury in riverine population from Madeira river basin. All the samples from Manicoré are male's hair.

The methylmercury levels in hair samples from Madeira river basin (Humaitá and Manicoré) presented lower average values, below 11.50 $mg.kg^{-1}$ and average percentages of methylmercury to total mercury (below 75%), than Tapajós river basin. These populations have a higher ingestion of a non-carnivorous fish. Very low percentage of MeHg (8.7%) was found in a goldminer (total Hg was 71.35 $mg.kg^{-1}$ and 6.20 $mg.kg^{-1}$ as MeHg) where main exposure is probably due to Hg^0

In other words, it can be ascertained that riverine populations are much more exposed to MeHg than goldminers. This is consistent with the dietary habits of the groups involved.

The samples, from Manicoré and Humaitá, collected at 1990, presented high average percentages of MeHg to total mercury (above 70%). Nevertheless the samples collected at the same places but in different periods, 1991 and 1992, showed percentages of MeHg below 70%. Probably these populations have consumed some fish less contaminated due to the fact that gold mining activity is decreasing in this river basin.

The total Hg results presented in the populations living on Madeira river basin are similar to the ones reported previously in Boischio *et al.* (1995)

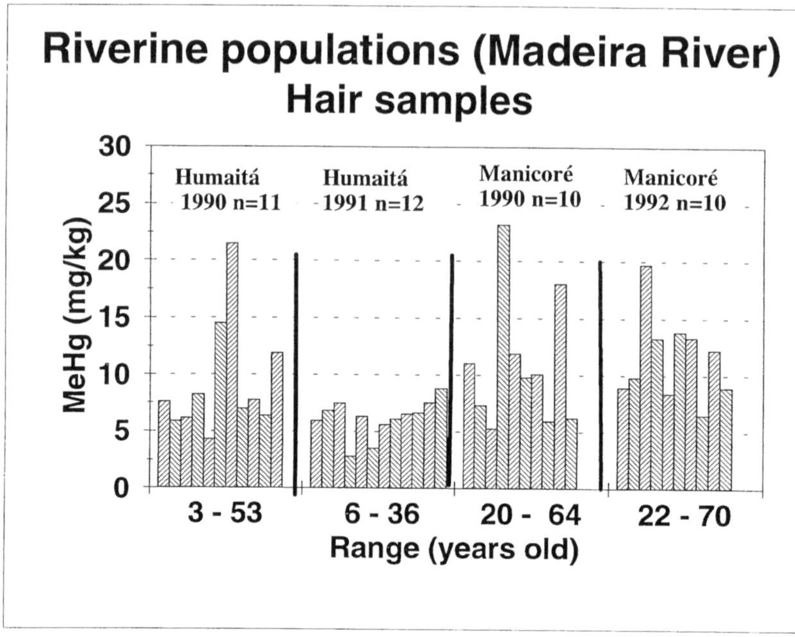

Figure 7 : Distribution of MeHg concentration in fishing village from Madeira river basin

The riverine population from some tributaries of Madeira river presented the highest averages of methylmercury values, above 20.00 mg.kg^{-1}. These exceptions, probably occur due to these populations only consume fish and fish productions. Their consumption of fish is around 7 times per week.

Figure 8 shows the distribution of methylmercury and percentages of methylmercury to total mercury in hair samples from one family. It is a riverine family from Machado river, one of the tributaries of Madeira river. All members of these family presented methylmercury concentration above 17.00 mg.kg^{-1}. Only the two young children with 14 months and two years old presented percentages of methylmercury below 40%, indicating contamination with inorganic and organic mercury. The others members present percentages above 70%, indicating that organic mercury was the predominant form of mercury in these hair samples.

In a study of Skerfving (1991), it was reported that the concentrations of total mercury in breast milk and in the blood plasma of breast-feeding infants were correlated to those in the maternal plasma. In our case, the mother of one family (Figure 9) was continuously exposed to methylmercury through fish consumption, and according to literature around 80% of mercury excreted in her breast milk to her infants was presented in the inorganic form, what probably justify the low levels of MeHg in the children.

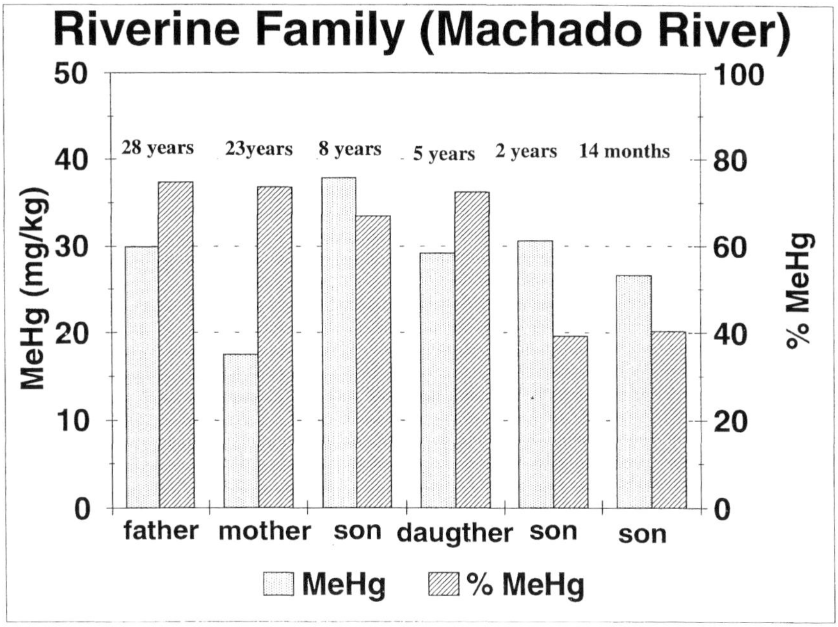

Figure 8: Distribution of MeHg levels and % MeHg from Madeira river tributary collected in June 1995

Figure 9 shows the results of a longitudinal analysis of mercury and methylmercury levels in the hair of the mother of the family. This young woman, during pregnancy was exposed to methylmercury (levels in hair above 18.00 $mg.kg^{-1}$). Babies born from mothers exposed to these levels of methylmercury, have a low risk, 5%, of neurological abnormalities (WHO, 1990). But her baby (14 months), which had high levels of methylmercury in his hair sample (Figure 8) did not present any evident neurotoxic effect of methylmercury. The highest MeHg levels occur in November, when the dry season was finishing. Seasonal variation was observed in fish from this area with the highest concentration at this same time (Malm *et al*, 1995).

The Yanomami Indians, which live in Roraima state in top north Brazilian Amazon, presented all the results of methylmercury levels in hair below the value of 6 $mg.kg^{-1}$(Figure 10). These results , probably occurred due to the fact that those Indians basic foods are wild animals, native and cultivated fruits and few fish (Castro *et al.*, 1991). Furthermore, we did not find any correlation between methylmercury concentrations and the sex of the Indians.

No clear relation was observed between MeHg levels and age in all Amazonians groups studied.

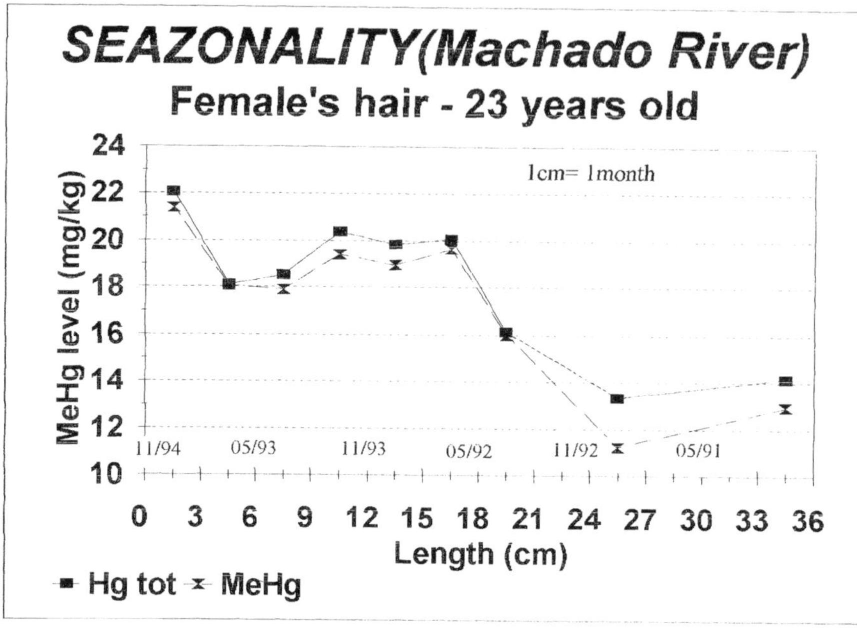

Figure 9: Longitudinal MeHg analysis along mother's hair strands sampled in November 1994

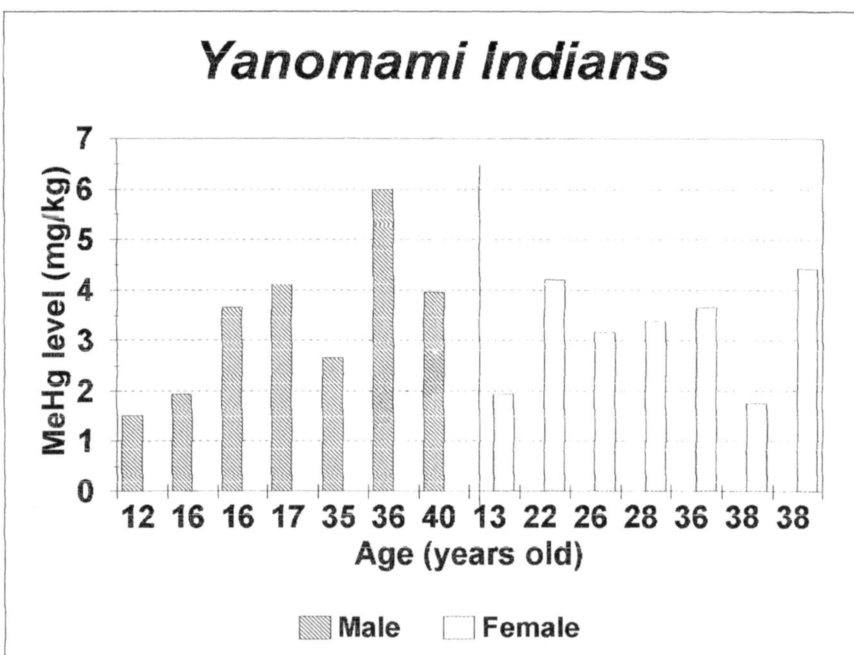

Figure 10: Distribution of MeHg in Yanomami Indians' hair collected in 1990

4. Conclusions

The applied methodology could be considered very efficient and at the same time extremely simple mainly regarding the extraction procedure.

A highly significant correlation was found in the interlaboratory exercise between National Institute for Minamata Disease and our laboratory at Federal University of Rio de Janeiro.

Precision and accuracy of analytical method were demonstrated with a comparison exercise with standard samples from IAEA.

In fishing villages and in riverine populations, the hair samples of inhabitants presented high percentages of MeHg to total Hg, indicating that methylmercury was the predominant form of mercury in hair samples and that people were mainly exposed to mercury through the consumption of contaminated fish with methylmercury. These clearly show the relationship between environmental contamination by mercury and dietary habits.

Seasonal variations in Amazon region can be expected in human hair methylmercury concentrations due to changing human fish diet along the year as well as seasonal variation of Hg in fish.

The most serious concern is regarding to women at child - bearing age due to the fact that most of results in this group are close to threshold levels of methylmercury concentrations in hair samples (above 10 $mg.kg^{-1}$.)

References

Airey, D.: 1983. *Environ. Health Perspect.* **52**: 303-316.

Akagi, H., Nishimura, H.: 1991. *Advances in mercury toxicology,* Plenum Press, New York, p. 53 - 76.

Akagi, H., Kinjo, Y, Branches, F.J.P., Malm, O., Harada, M., Pfeiffer, W.C., Kato, H.: 1994. *Environmental Sciences,* **3**(1): 25 - 32.

Akagi, H., Malm, O., Branches, F. J. P., Kinjo, Y., Kashima, Y., Guimarães, J. R. D., Oliveira, R. B., Haraguchi, K., Pfeiffer, W. C., Takizawa, Y., Kato, H.: 1995a. *Water, Air, and Soil Pollution* **80**: 85 - 94.

Akagi, H., Malm, O., Kinjo, Y., Harada, M., Branches, F. J. P., Pfeiffer, W. C., Kato, H.: 1995b. *Sci Total Environ.***175**: 85-95.

Boischio, A. A., Heenshel, D., Barbosa, A. C.:1995. *Ecosystem Health* **1**(3):177-192.

Canner, P., Clarkson, T. W., Nordberg, G.: 1979. *Handbook on the Toxicology of Metals.* Elsevier/ North-Holland Biomedical Press, Amsterdan, Holland, p. 65-97.

Castro, M. B., Albert, B., Pfeiffer, W. C.: 1991. Proc. 8th Int. Conf. Heavy Metals in the Environ., Edinburgh, p. 367 - 370.

Clarkson, T. W.: 1989. *Journal of American College of Toxicology*.**8**: 1291-1295.

Choi, B.H.: 1989. *Progress in Neurobiology* 32: 447 - 470.

Cox, C., Clarkson, T.W., Marsh, D.O., Amin - Zaki, L., Tikriti, S., Myers, G.G.: 1989. *Environ. Res.*, **49:** 318 - 332.

Girard, M., Dumont, C.: 1995. *Water, Air, and Soil Pollution* **80**: 13 - 19.

Guimarães, J. R. D; Malm, O., Pfeiffer, W.C.: 1995. *Sci. Total Environ.* **175**(2) 151-162.

Lebel, J., Mergler, D., Lucotte, M., Amorim, M., Dolbec, J., Miranda, D., Arantes, G., Rheault, I., Picchet, P.: 1996. *Neuro Toxicology* **17**(1): 157-168.

Lindqvist, O Jernelov, A Johansson, K and Rodhe, H.: 1984: Report PM1816, National Swedish Protection Board, Solna, Sweden.

Malm, O., Pfeiffer, W.C., Souza, C.M.M., Reuther, R.: 1990. *AMBIO* **19**, 11 - 15.

Malm, O., Castro, M.B.; Bastos, W.R.; Branches, F.J.P.; Guimarães, J.R.D.; Zuffo, C.E., and Pfeiffer, W.C.: 1995. *Sci. Total Environ.* **175**(2) 127-140

Malm, O.; Guimarães, JRD; Castro, MB; Bastos, WR; Viana, JP and Pfeiffer, WC. 1995.. Proceedings of the International Symposiumon Mercury in the Environment: Low level Exposure and its Potential Effects on Man. Nov., 16. Kumamoto, Japan. pp. 44-50.

Skerfving, S.: 1991. *Bull. Environ.Contam. Toxicol.*, **46**: 255.

Tsubaki, T., Takahashi, H.: 1986. Minamata Disease Studies, KODANSHA LTD, Tokyo, Japan, p. 41 - 132.

WHO: 1976. IPCS - *Mercury* Criteria 1

WHO: 1990. IPCS - *Methylmercury - Environmental Health* Criteria 101.

FISH DIET AND MERCURY EXPOSURE IN A RIPARIAN AMAZONIAN POPULATION

J. LEBEL[1], M. ROULET[2], D. MERGLER[1], M. LUCOTTE[2] and F. LARRIBE[1]

[1]*Centre pour l'étude des interactions biologiques entre la santé et l'environnement (CINBIOSE), Université du Québec à Montréal, Succ. Centre-Ville, Montréal, Canada, H3C 3P8.* [2]*Chaire de recherche en environnement Hydro-Québec/CRSNG/UQAM, Montréal, Canada.*

Abstract. The incorporation of mercury into the food chain and its assimilation by humans is a universally recognized potential health hazard. Studies carried out in the Amazon Basin have shown that mercury (Hg) is present in fish and in humans, however, the relation between fish diet and human exposure has received limited attention in this region. The present study focused on a small village, Brasília Legal (3°59'00"S, 55°30'00"W), situated on the banks of the Rio Tapajós. A total of 181 fish (40 species) were captured in March, 1995 and analysed for Hg concentration. Of these, 132 fish were among species consumed by the population during the rainy season (mid-November to mid-May) and the dry season (mid-May to mid-November). Wide intra- and inter-species variations in Hg concentrations were observed. Thirty four fish (25.8% of the consumed species) had levels above 0.5 μg/g Hg fresh weight; all were among the piscivorous and omnivorous species. Hair Hg concentrations (HHg), showed that villagers with a high fish diet (n=31; median HHg=16.1 μg/g) and mixed fish diet (n=36; median HHg=14.8 μg/g) had significantly higher HHg concentrations compared to the low fish diet group (n=29; mean HHg=7.8 μg/g). Time series function of HHg measurements, made for 26 persons with over 24 cm of hair, revealed sinusoidal variations, with peaks during the rainy season and troughs during the low water period, paralleling the seasonal shift in dietary habits. Piscivorous and omnivorous fish species, with higher mercury levels, are the main component of the fish diet during the rainy season, while herbivorous fish species predominate during the dry season. Preventive actions should take into account the risk to human health, particularly for fetal and neonatal development, the importance of fish in the riparian diet, the wide intra- and inter -species variations in mercury content and seasonal fluctuations in diet.

1. Introduction

The incorporation of mercury into the food chain and its assimilation by humans is a universally recognized potential health hazard. When mercury is released into aquatic environments, it can be methylated by bacteria, present in river sediments, to its organic form: methylmercury. In this form, it then becomes bioavailable to the ichthyofauna, where it can be biomagnified through every step of the food chain up to humans (WHO, 1989). In areas where fish are highly contaminated by mercury, populations, who frequently consume these fish, are at risk for neurotoxic and teratogenic damage, resulting from mercury poisoning (WHO, 1990).

Since the late eighties, numerous studies have reported the presence of mercury in different compartments of the Amazon Basin ecosystem. Two mercury sources appear to be implicated in this contamination: gold mining activities (Martinelli *et al.*, 1988; Malm *et al.*, 1990; Lacerda and Salomons, 1991; Pfeiffer *et al.*, 1991; Pfeiffer *et al.*, 1993) and slash and burn agricultural practices resulting in lixiviation of soils, loaded with natural mercury, to the aquatic system (Roulet *et al.*, 1996a,1996b). The studies on mercury content of fish in the Amazonian river system have shown that levels often surpass 0.5 μg/g fresh weight (Pfeiffer *et al.*, 1991; Lacerda and Salomons, 1991; Barbosa *et al.*, 1995; Boischio *et al.*, 1995; Malm *et al.*, 1995a), a value that is considered in many countries as a standard not to be exceeded for safe consumption.

Hair mercury levels, assessed in human populations living in various areas of the Brazilian Amazon, are in the range of a few μg/g up to 300 μg/g, with median exposure values in the order of 2 μg/g up to ± 20 μg/g (Akagi *et al.*, 1995; Malm *et al.*, 1995b; Barbosa *et al.*, 1995; Boischio *et al.*, 1995; Grandjean *et al.*, 1993; Nakanishi, 1992;

Lebel *et al.,* 1996; Boischio *et al.,* 1996). Even if many of these studies report results from small, heterogeneous samples, the general conclusion is that methylmercury exposure in the Amazon could present a risk for the health of these populations.

The toxic effects of methylmercury were dramatically brought to light following the Minamata and Niigata poisonings. In these disasters, consumption of highly contaminated fish by the local population, over a short period of time (few months), resulted in high exposure levels (> 50 µg/g Hg in hair), followed by the apparition of a neurologic syndrome and teratogenic damage, later called Minamata Disease (WHO, 1976; WHO, 1990). The exposure profile in the Amazon is different. Low-level methylmercury has probably been present for at least 20 years, when gold mining activities started and possibly as long as 40 years, with the introduction of slash and burn activities (Roulet *et al.*, 1996a, 1996b). Recent investigations of communities living on the banks of the Tapajós River have shown dose-related nervous system dysfunction, in the absence of classic Minamata disease symptomatology (Lebel *et al.*, 1996).

Although there is information from the Amazon Basin on mercury levels in fish and in humans, the relation between fish diet and exposure has received limited attention. The Amazonian environment is complex: there is great biodiversity, extreme climatic conditions (high temperature and humidity with important precipitation) and seasonal fluctuations of the water levels that can reach a difference of 6 meters between the rainy season (Mid-November to Mid-May) and the dry season (Mid-May to Mid-November). These characteristics greatly influence fish behaviour and the availability of fish ressources (Goulding, 1980).

The objective of the present study was to characterize methyl mercury exposure of a riparian population in the Amazon Basin by: i) determining mercury concentration in a large sample of fish from their fishing grounds ii) surveying fish consumption during the rainy and dry season, and iii) examining hair mercury concentration with respect to diet and over time.

2. Materials and Methods

STUDY SITE. The study focused on a small village, Brasília Legal (3°59'00"S, 55°30'00"W), situated on the banks of the Rio Tapajós, a main tributary of the Amazon River. The village is approximately 250 km downstream from the most extensive currently operated gold-mining fields in Brazil (Malm *et al.,* 1995b) and in the midst of extensively deforestated river banks. Brasília Legal is accessible only by water, a 12-18 hour boat trip from Santarém, a city of three hundred thousand. The villagers are not exposed to mercury vapours.

FISH COLLECTION AND ANALYSIS. Fish were collected in March 1995 at 16 sites within a 1 km radius of Brasília Legal at sites identified by local fishermen as commonly used for their fishing activities. Sample collection was done using the same type of fish nets as the local fishermen. The nets were 20 m long with mesh size of 40 mm x 40 mm. Fishing activities were conducted between 5:00 AM and 10:00 PM with collections in the morning, noon and night.

Immediate identification of fish was done with a taxonomic key and with the help of fishermen. Weight, length, sex determination, and stomach content analyses were performed on every captured fish. A piece of muscle tissue, without the skin, was taken laterally, below the dorsal fin and frozen individually in polyethylene vials for future mercury analysis. Total mercury analyses were performed in the laboratories of the

Environmental Research Chair of the University of Québec in Montréal, using Cold Vapour Atomic Fluorescence spectrophotometry (CVAF) according to the method described by Plourde *et al.*, (1996).

POPULATION AND DIET CHARACTERIZATION. Participants were recruited throughout the village. During the third week of March 1995 (rainy season), a total of 96 persons (46 women and 50 men), representing 39.7% of the adult population (≥15 years old) of 242 inhabitants responded to an interview-administrated questionnaire on the previous 5 days' diet. For each day, they indicated the number of meals, whether or not they had eaten fish during this meal and identified the type of fish at each fish meal. A second survey was done in the first week of November, 1995 (end of the dry season), at which time the questionnaire was re-administered to 79 of the original participants (82.3%).

HAIR ANALYSIS. In March, 1995, a hair strand, from each participant, was collected from the root in the occipital region and then placed in plastic bags, with the root end stapled. Mercury analyses were conducted in the laboratories of the Environmental Research Chair of the University of Québec in Montréal, using Cold Vapour Atomic Fluorescence spectrophotometry (CVAF).

Hair strands were cut in one cm segments and each segment (up to 24) was analysed for total mercury, according to the procedure described by Bloom and Fitzgerald (1988) and adapted for hair digestion. The segmental analysis of hair provides the opportunity to reconstitute past exposure history since hair growth rate is approximately 1 cm per month (Clarkson *et al.*, 1988; Cernichiari *et al.*, 1995). Inorganic mercury determination was done on the first segment using the methods described by Farant *et al.*, (1981) and adapted for CVAF. Analytical quality was ensured by including a Health Canada sample of powdered hair in the series. Methylmercury was calculated for the first cm of hair, as the difference between total mercury and inorganic mercury. Mean mercury hair level (HHg) was determined for each person by averaging the mercury concentrations measured in each centimeter.

STATISTICAL ANALYSIS. Descriptive statistics are used to illustrate mercury concentration in fish and to characterize fish diet. Mean comparisons were carried out using ANOVA with Tukey post-hoc analysis for inter-group differences or where necessary, non-parametric tests of comparison (Mann Whitney, Kruskall Wallis). The chronological sequence of hair mercury levels were described using a polynomial regression model and the sinusoidal variations were confirmed with sample autocorrelation function. The autocorrelation coefficient is a measure of the linear dependance in the observations separated by time periods. If adjacent observations (one time periods apart) tend to move together, then $r_1 > 0$, while if observations two time periods apart tend to move in opposite directions then $r_2 < 0$ and so forth (Box and Jenkins, 1970). All analyses were performed using the *SAS* statistical package.

3. Results

Table I contains a list of the 40 species (181 fish) that were captured in March, 1995. The most frequently captured fish were: Aracu (43 individuals), Pescada (39 individuals), Piranha (29 individuals), and Caratinga (14 individuals), which made up 72.9% of the total captures. The feeding habits, determined for each individual from the

TABLE I

Mercury concentration in fish captured in the Rio Tapajós, Brasília Legal Area, March, 1995.

SPECIES	(n)	Feeding habits[1]	Mean Hg (µg/g fresh weight)	Standard deviation	Minimum and Maximum values
Acari sp.	3	B	0.03	0.01	0.03-0.04
Acari pedra	1	B	0.05		
Apapa amarelo	2	P	0.61	0.06	0.57-0.65
Apapa branco	4	P	0.54	0.09	0.42-0.62
Aracu amarelo	4	H	0.11	0.05	0.04-0.16
Aracu comun	32	H	0.08	0.08	0.03-0.37
Aracu cabeça gordo	7	H	0.33	0.47	0.05-1.34
Barbado	1	P	0.28		
Caratinga	14	H	0.09	0.04	0.03-0.19
Carauacu	1	O	0.17		
Curivina	1	B	0.10		
Dourada	1	P	0.31		
Filhote	4	P	0.53	0.18	0.38-0.79
Jacunda	1	P	0.27		
Jiju	1	P	0.38		
Mapara	1	H	0.26		
Mandi	2	P	0.30	0.06	0.26-0.35
Mandube	1	O	0.40		
Mocinha	2	B	0.18	0.12	0.10-0.27
Pacu sp.	5	H	0.04	0.02	0.01-0.06
Pacu manteiga	1	H	0.02		
Pacu marreca	1	H	0.03		
Peixe cachorro	1	P	0.52		
Pescada branca	36	P	0.53	0.23	0.13-1.35
Pescada pitinga	1	H	0.06		
Pescada vermelha	2	H	0.10	0.01	0.09-0.11
Piracatinga	2	P	0.76	0.19	0.62-0.89
Pirarucu	1	P	0.17		
Piranha branca	11	0	0.53	0.31	0.07-1.12
Piranha caju	5	P	0.55	0.12	0.41-0.67
Piranha mafura	1	P	0.09		
Piranha mucura	1	P	0.13		
Piranha preta	11	O	0.40	0.13	0.09-0.59
Saranha	2	O	0.37	0.08	0.31-0.42
Sarda	2	P	0.80	0.38	0.53-1.07
Sardinha	6	O	0.13	0.10	0.02-0.30
Surubim	1	P	0.36		
Tambaqui	1	F	0.07		
Traira	1	P	0.49		
Tucunare	6	P	0.40	0.19	0.21-0.75

[1]B: Benthonophage; P: Piscivorous; H: Herbivorous; O: Omnivorous; F: Frugivorous

stomach content analysis or literature review when the stomach was empty, were distributed in the following manner: piscivorous (n=73 (40.3%)), herbivorous (n=68 (37.6%)), omnivorous (n=32 (17.7%)), benthonophage (n=7 (3.9%)) and frugivorous (n=1 (0.5%)). Mean mercury concentration varied from 0.02 μg/g fresh weight for Pacu manteiga, up to 0.80 μg/g fresh weight ± 0.38 for Sarda. It is noteworthy that for certain species for which there is information on a large number of individuals, there is a fairly large range of mercury content. For example, for Pescada branca, levels range from 0.13 μg/g fresh weight to 1.35 μg/g fresh weight.

Figure 1 shows the percentile distribution of mercury concentration for the piscivorous, omnivorous and herbivorous fish species consumed by the local population in March, 1995. The mean values for the 3 categories are 0. 51± 0.22 μg/g fresh weight, 0.46 ± 0.24 μg/g fresh weight and 0.07± 0.07 μg/g fresh weight, respectively. The latter group is significantly lower than the two others (Tukey post hoc; $p<0.0001$). A total of 34 individual fish (25.8%) had mercury concentrations above 0.5 μg/g fresh weight; 26 of these were piscivorous, representing 45.6% of all of the piscivorous fish, and 8 were omnivorous, representing 36.3% of all of the omnivorous fish.

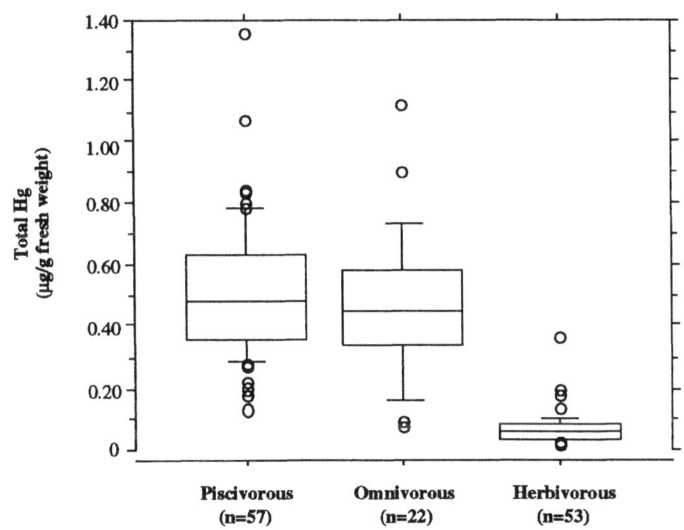

Fig. 1. Percentile distribution of Hg concentrations in piscivorous, omnivorous and herbivorous fish species, captured in March 1995, and consumed by the local population. The mid line of the box plot indicates the median, the upper and lower lines of the box indicate the 75th and 25th percentile, respectively; the upper and lower lines indicate the 90th and 10th percentile and the circles are above and below these levels.

In the diet survey covering 5 days in March, during the rainy season, fish meals constituted an average of 47.9% ± 34.2%; of the total meals eaten (median: 57.8%), ranging from none to 100%. For the meals surveyed in November 1995 (end of dry season), the villagers reported that fish meals made up on average 45.2% ± 30.2 (median: 50.0%) of their meals, ranging from none to 100%. The non-fish meals consisted of beans, eggs, poultry or meat.

Figure 2 presents the distribution of HHg for the entire population. The median value was 12.9μg/g. Men had significantly higher HHg levels (median 15.7μg/g) than women (median 11.2μg/g) (Mann Whitney; $p<0.02$). However, these differences could be attributed to the fishermen (n=14), whose median HHg concentration, 27.3 μg/g, was significantly higher (Kruskal-Wallis; $p<0.001$) than the other men (median 12.2μg/g) and the women. These differences are likewise reflected in fish consumption during the rainy season; the fishermen ate on an average 68.8% ± 28.8 fish meals, while for the rest of the population, it was 43.9% ± 33.6 for men, and 44.7% ± 34.6 for women.

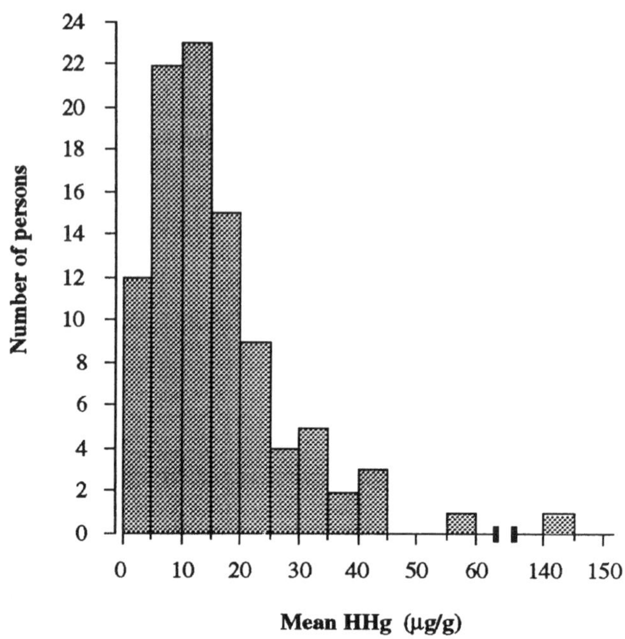

Fig. 2. Distribution of mean hair Hg (HHg) concentrations for villagers of Brasilia Legal (n = 96).

No relation was observed between HHg and age, however the persons with the highest educational level (≥ 6 years) had signficantly lower concentrations as compared to the others (medians: 15.2 μg/g vs 9.8 μg/g; Mann-Whitney; $p<0.02$). For the entire group, methylmercury constitued an average of 89.6% ± 3.0% of the total hair Hg, with a minimum value of 72.8% and a maximum of 93.6%.

The population was categorized according to their fish consumption in the rainy season. Those whose fish meals made up 75% or more of their total meals, were classified "high fish diet", those whose fish meals made up 25% - 75% of their total meals, were classifed "mixed diet", while those with less than 25% fish meals, were considered "low fish diet". HHg percentile distributions of mean hair mercury level (HHg) for these three groups are presented in Figure 3. The two outliers, whose HHg are 142.4 μg/g and 59.4 μg/g, respectively, were fishermen, although the latter had done little fishing during the week of the survey. These outliers were excluded for the group comparisons, which revealed that those with a low fish diet had significantly less hair mercury content as compared to the two others (Tukey post hoc; $p<0.001$).

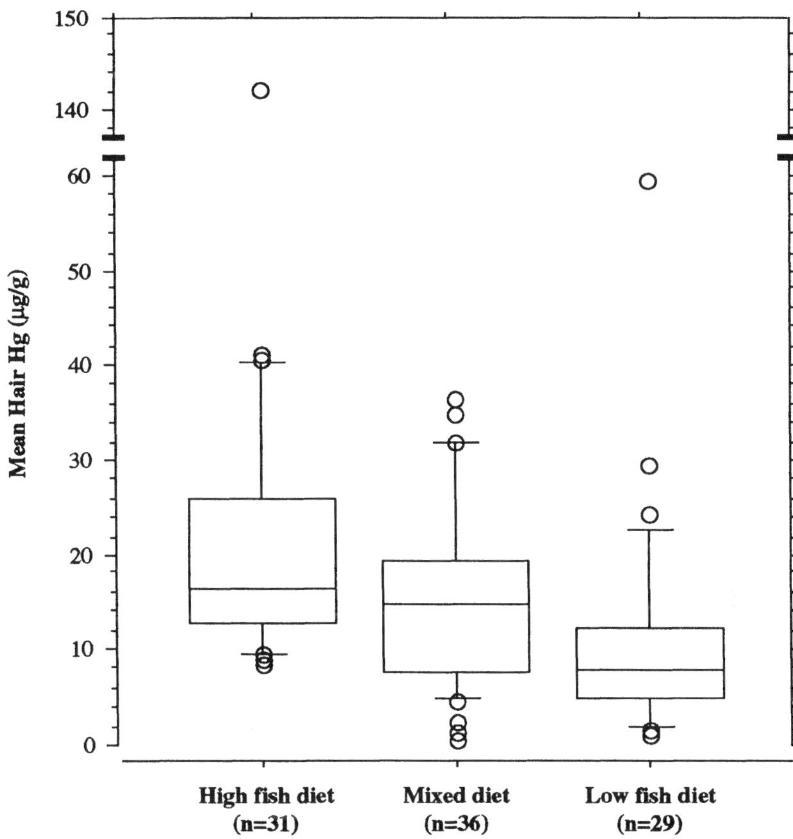

Fig. 3. Percentile distribution of HHg concentrations for villagers with high fish diet (> 75% fish meals), mixed diet (≥ 25 < 75% fish meals) and low fish diet (<25% fish meals). The mid line of the box plot indicates the median, the upper and lower lines of the box indicate the 75th and 25th percentile; the upper and lower lines indicate the 90th and 10th percentile and the circles are above and below these levels.

The distribution of fish species over all of the meals is presented in Figure 4, which shows the relative frequency of fish species consumption, calculated as the percentage of all meals of a particular fish species over the total meals for the week surveyed. It can be seen that in the high water season, Pescada, a piscivorous fish was the fish most frequently eaten, while in the low water season, it was Pacu, a herbivorous fish. Overall, piscivorous and omnivorous fish constituted 36.2% of the meals in the rainy season, while herbivourous fish made up 11.9% of the meals. At the end of the dry season these percentages were inversed: 11.0% for piscivorous and omnivorous fish and 33.7% for herbivorous fish.

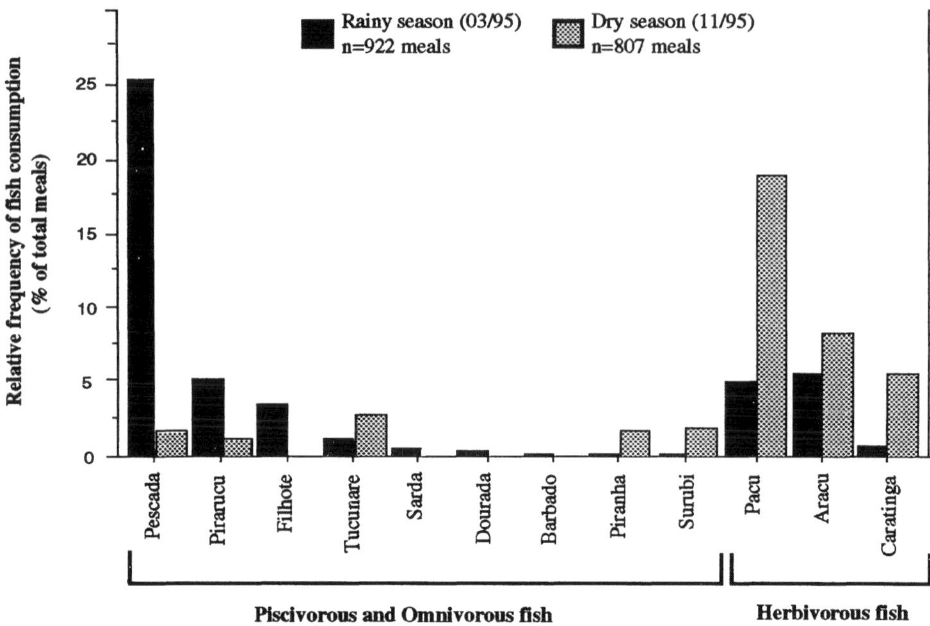

Fig. 4. Relative frequency of fish meals of a particular species with respect to the total number of meals over a five day period in the rainy (March 1995) and dry (November 1995) seasons.

Sequential hair analyses were used to examine the Hg variations over time. All persons had at least 2 cm, however, the total number of centimeters was signficantly less for men as compared to women. The longest hair for men was 9 cm, while 26 women had a minimum of 24 cm. Thus, in order to examine sequential segmental variations, only the women with 24 centimeters, representing approximately 2 years of exposure, were included. Figure 5 shows the mean profile of segmental hair mercury concentrations for these women. The value from the first centimeter was assigned to the beginning of March 1995 since growth of the hair follicle to the midpoint of the first cm takes approximately 20 days (Hislop et al., 1983) and we collected hair during the third week of March. The levels vary in a sinusoidal fashion, with the highest concentrations in the 1st and the 12th centimeter and the lowest at the 7th and the 19th centimeter, which if one considers hair growth at approximately 1 cm/mo, the high levels would correspond to March 1995 and March 1994 and the low concentrations to August 1994 and August 1993. Thus, the peaks would occur during the rainy season, while the troughs during the dry season. The differences between the peaks and the troughs are significant for the two years (Wilcoxon Signed Rank: $p<0.05$). The variations over time can best be approximated by a 6th order polynomial regression.

To confirm the seasonality of the time series, we submitted the data to sample auto-correlation function; the results are presented in Fig 6. The auto-correlation varies sinusoidally around zero, with positive values from the 1st to 5th centimeter, and the 11th

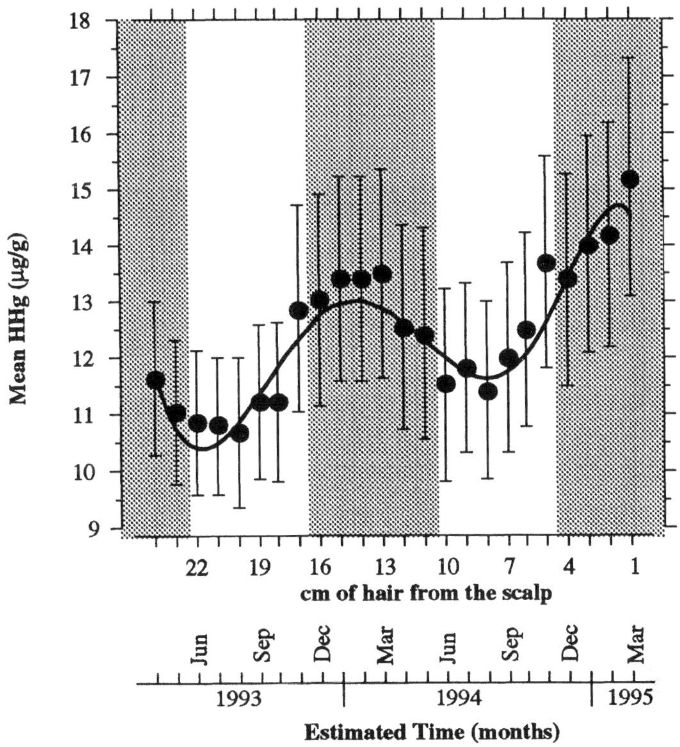

Fig. 5. HHg variation over 24 centimeters for the 26 women with sufficient hair strands. The time (in months) is based on estimated hair growth of 1 cm/month. Vertical bars represent ± 1 standard error. The line of best fit, a 6th order polynomial is illustrated. Shaded areas represent the rainy season; the unshaded portions correspond to the dry season.

to 15th centimeter, and negative values over the 6th to 10th centimeter and the 16th to 23rd centimeter. This profile, with large opposing values at r6 and r12 is typical of seasonal fluctuations (Chatfield, 1984)

4. Discussion

The large sample of fish, taken from the Tapajós River, within a radius of 1 km from the village, Brasília Legal, using nets similar to those of the local fishermen, provides an important data set on the icthyofauna, which form the basis of the villagers' diet. The important biodiversity of this limited area was reflected by the capture of forty different fish species from five different trophic levels. The results of the mercury analysis revealed wide intra- and inter-species variations, although the highest levels were observed in the piscivorous and omnivorous fish. As expected, it is within these groups that the fish with mercury concentrations above 0.5 μg/g fresh weight were encountered.

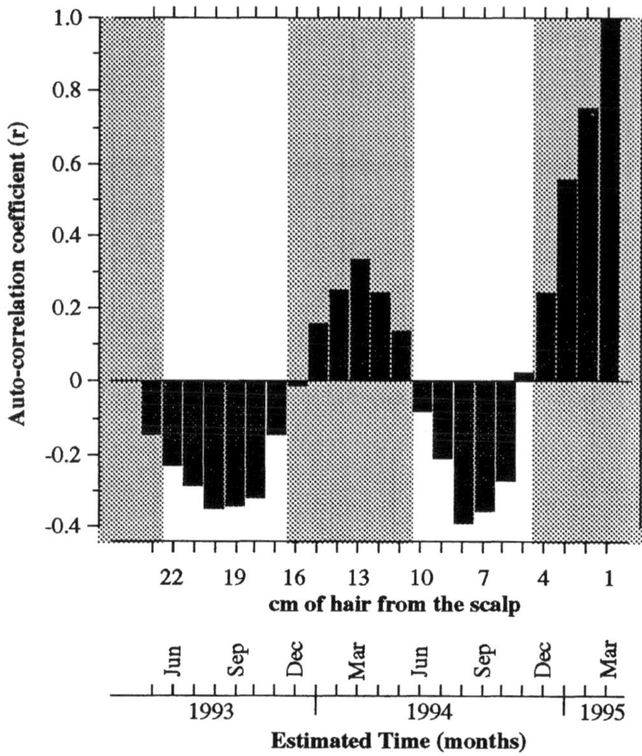

Fig. 6. Sample autocorrelation function for the HHg 24 cm time series for 26 women's hair strands. The ordinate is the autocorrelation coefficient (r) and the abscissa is in centimeters of hair. . The time (in months) is based on estimated hair growth of 1 cm/month. Shaded areas represent the rainy season; the unshaded portions correspond to the dry season.

Although this type of sampling strategy differs from previous studies in the area where small numbers of fish were collected in a wide variety of areas through fishing or from marketplaces (Malm *et al.*, 1995b; Boischio *et al.*, 1995), fish mercury content is within a similar range.

The relation between fish weight and mercury concentration was not presented because we believe that a different study design and data set is required to perform these analyses. Such a size selective study would be long term, with nets of different mesh size in order to capture fish of different length and weight, over an extended period of time. In the present study, we primarly focused our attention on collecting the typical catch, consumed by the population. It is true that the information gathered here does not provide the opportunity to say if small fish are less contaminated than big fish, but it gives the importance of the contamination of the fish that are eaten.

Due to the considerable long half life (months to years) of methylmercury in fish, reported for species in different environments (Lockhart *et al.*, 1972; WHO, 1989), we can presume that the mercury concentrations found in the fish from the Rio Tapajós captured during the rainy season would not be very different from the concentrations that would be encountered in the following dry season. Moreover, seasonal variability is probably inferior to intra-species variability, which was, for many species, very important. This assumption of the relative stability of mercury in fish, served as the basis for the interpretation of the variations in hair mercury concentrations over time in relation to diet. This is currently being investigated by our group with a sample of fish collected during the dry period.

In this village of the Amazon Basin, where fish is a dietary mainstay, hair mercury levels appear to vary sinusoidally over time, paralleling the seasonal variations in fish species consumption during the rainy and dry seasons. Proportionally more pisciverous fish are eaten in the rainy season, while in the dry season, more herbivorous fish are consumed. This probably reflects fish bioavailability due to differences in the life cycle characteristics of the various species. The piscivorous and omnivorous fish with higher mercury concentrations than the herbivorous species would account for the important rise in hair mercury during the rainy period followed by a decreasing trend, corresponding to the consumption of herbivorous fish species with lower mercury levels, during the dry period. The correspondence between the fluctuations in HHg and seasonal variations in water level is based on the assumption that hair growth is approximately 1 cm per month. Although it has been suggested that hair growth may be more or less rapid and, of course, every month does not have the same number of days (Cernichiari *et al.*, 1995), the picture would not differ dramatically taking these factors into account. The fluctuations in HHg cannot be attributed to diminished or increased fish consumption during one of these periods since the relative frequency of fish meals over the entire diet is similar for both seasons, constituting approximately half of the meals.

Since only women had hair lengths greater than 24 cm, their hair strands were used to illustrate variations over time, providing a comparable data set. Had we included the entire population in the analyses, those with short hair, in particular fishermen, a group with higher HHg concentrations would have raised the first portion of the seasonal profile, providing an erroneous picture of the trend. Indeed, the curve would had shown an important increase in HHg during the last months of 1994 and the first of 1995. The approach taken here, in evaluating the seasonal pattern, allows us to extrapolate the general trend encountered in these women to the entire population. One should be very careful in affirming increases or decreases in exposure from point samples since both fish diet and time of the year appear to affect mercury hair concentrations .

The seasonal variation in fish consumption was surveyed for a one-week period in order to obtain information on fish-eating habits in both seasons. It should be noted that all the fish consumed in one or the other season were among those that were captured in March, 1995. Thus, the fact that we only analyzed mercury levels for fish captured in the rainy period does not limit the interpretations on seasonal fluctuations. The use of an interview administered diet questionnaire allowed us to gather precise, species-specific data, and standardize fish consumption in terms of numbers of meals. There are, however, drawbacks. First, it is based on the assumption that the surveyed week corresponds to the entire season; it is always possible that in this particular week, food consumption was distributed differently from the other weeks. Nevertheless, collective discussion with the population confirmed that Pescada was indeed the most frequently consumed fish during the rainy season, while Pacu and Aracu were the fish most frequently eaten during the dry season. Second, the dietary survey used in this study did not take into account the quantity of fish eaten at each meal, thereby increasing inter-individual variability. Moreover, we did not have a measure of the actual amount of mercury ingested per meal, as has been done in other studies (Boischio *et al.*, 1995; 1996). The method used here did allow us to classify persons according to their dietary pattern into high, mixed and low fish diets, which were reflected by hair mercury levels.

As has been noted in previous studies in this region (Boischio *et al.*, 1995; 1996; Malm *et al.*, 1995b; Lebel *et al.*, 1996), many of the villagers had HHg levels considerably higher than those that are thought to produce deleterious effects on the foetus, that is, peak maternal hair concentrations of 10 µg/g to 20 µg/g (WHO, 1990). Moreover, dose-related nervous system dysfunction has been observed in young adults in this population (Lebel *et al.*, 1996). These results suggest that methylmercury exposure in this area is adversely affecting the health and well-being of this population.

It is interesting to note that those with the highest level of education had significantly lower levels of hair mercury. Over the past 6 years, there have been a fair number of visits to this community by Brazilian and foreign researchers, seeking information on mercury contamination. These visits, coupled to discussions with the local population, have created a growing awareness of the potential danger of methylmercury consumption, particularly through piscivorous and omnivorous fish. The lower hair mercury concentrations among the most educated persons possibly reflects this awareness.

This observation should be taken into consideration for future development and implementation of preventive measures that would help to reduce the body burden of mercury resulting from the consumption of contaminated fish. In a population where fish is such an important food source, arguing for a complete ban of fish consumption is illusory and would most probably have a deleterious health impact. On the other hand, development of a program based on a *black list* of fish species not to be eaten remains equivocal since the wide intra-species variation in Hg concentration for many fish species is important. The range of concentrations for a single species is often distributed on both sides of the standard set in Brazil (0.5 µg/g fresh weight) for safe consumption of fish (Brasil, Ministerio da Saude, 1975). Therefore, putting a proscription on a particular fish species could result in the prohibition of consumption of fish that in many cases could be eaten.

The development of a perfect mitigation measure in this situation is difficult. Our group's approach is oriented towards education and participation of the population in the understanding of the situation and the development of applicable measures for reduction of mercury exposure. Reducing exposure by dramatically changing the dietary habits that have been present for decades in a population, is difficult to achieve and was indicated as not being acceptable through discussion with the villagers. The short term measure that is favoured is a situation where all fish can be eaten, but where diet is directed towards a more frequent consumption of less contaminated fish, like the herbivorous species. The efficiency of this measure in terms of reduction of mercury exposure will need further investigation. Working with the population is a key element for appropriate implementation. As an example, the last morning we were in Brasília Legal, the teachers invited us to address the students to stimulate them to say in school and to explain the study. « Where is the mercury? » we ask. « In the fish » they answer. « And what can we do » « Eat more fish that don't eat other fish » they chant.

Acknowledgements

This project could not have taken place without the steadfast collaboration of Dr. Cristovan Waverly Diniz, pro-rector of the Federal University of Pará (UFPa), Sr. Aldo Queiroz Gomes, director of the UFPa-Santarém Campus, Dr. Marúcia Amorim of UFPa and Dr. Jean-Rémy Guimarães of the Federal University of Rio de Janeiro. Our field work was greatly facilitated due to the logistic coordination and diet questionnaire administration done by Sr. Umberto Da Silva from UFPa. Long hours of fish collection, identification, and dissection, were made easier with the help of Carlos José Sousa Passos, Gilbson Santos Soares, Erinaldo de Jesus da Silva, Luciana Silva da Costa, Ynglea Georgina de Freitos Goch, Heron Coelho, and Gil Seriques; all students in the environmental science program at UFPa-Santarém Campus or members of the NGO Amazonian Defense Group. We thank the staff of UFPa-Santarém Campus for their hospitality. Ms Julie Dolbec provided inestimable laboratory expertise in fish and hair analysis. Finally, we would like to express our gratitude to the population of Brasília Legal for their invaluable participation and collaboration in the accomplishment of this work. This study was financially supported by the International Development Research Centre (IDRC) of Canada (grant #96-1052-01/001300-01).

References

Akagi, H.,Malm, O., Kinjo, Y., Harada, M., Branches, F.P.J., Pfeiffer, W.C., and Kato, H.: 1995, *Sci. Total Environ.* **175**, 85-95.

Barbosa, A.C., Boischio, A.A., East, G.A., Ferrari, I., Gonçalvez, A., Silva, P.R.M., and Da Cruz, T.M.E.: 1995, *Water, Air and Soil Pollut.* **80**, 109-121.

Bloom, N., and Fitzgerald, W.F.: 1988, *Analytica Chimica Acta* **208**, 151-161.

Boischio, A.A.P., Henschel, D., and Barbosa, A.C.: 1995, *Ecosystem Health* **1**(3), 177-192.

Boischio, A.A.P., and Henschel, D.S.: 1996, *NeuroToxicology* **17**(1), 169-176.

Box, G.E.P., and Jenkins, G.M.: 1970, *Time Series Analysis: Forecasting and Control*, Holden-Day, San Francisco, California.

Brasil, Ministerio da Saude: 1975, *Resoluçao No. 18/75 da Commissao Nacional de Normas e Padroes Pará Alimentos. Diario oficial da Uniao, Brasília, 9 de Dezembro de 1975. Seçao 1*, p.16378.

Cernichiari, E., Toribaba, T.Y., Liang, L., Marsh, D.O., Berlin, M., Myers, G.J., Cox, C., Shamlaye, C.F., Choisy, O., Davidson, P.W., and Clarkson, T.W.: 1995, *NeuroToxicology* **16**(4), 613-628.

Chatfield, C.: 1984, *The analysis of time series: An Introduction*, Chapman and Hall, London, New-York.

Clarkson, T.W., Hursh, J.B., Sager, P.R., and Syversen, T.L.M.: 1988, In: Clarkson, T.W., Friberg, L., Nordberg, G.F., Sager, P. (editors). *Biological Monitoring of Metals*, Plenum Press, New-York, p. 199-246.

Farant, J.P., Brisset, D., Moncion, L., Bigras, L., and Chartrand, A.: 1981, *J. Anal. Toxicol.* **5**, 47-51.

Grandjean, P., Cardoso, B., and Guimares, G.: 1993, *Lancet* **342**, 991.

Goulding, M.,: 1980, *The fishes and the forest, explorations in Amazonian natural history*, University of California Press, Berkeley and Los Angeles, California, p. 1-9.

Hislop, J.S., Collier, T.R., White, G.P., Khatiny, D.T., and French, E.: 1983, In: Brown, S.S. (editors). *Clinical Toxicology and Clinical Chemistry of Metals*, Academic Press, New-York, p. 145-149.

Lacerda, L.D., and Salomons, W.: 1991, *Mercury in the Amazon: a chemical timebomb?* Report sponsored by the Dutch Ministry of Housing, Physical Planning and Environment, Chemical Timebomb Project.

Lebel. J., Mergler, D., Lucotte, M., Amorim, M., Dolbec, J., Miranda, D., Arantès, G., Rheault, I., and Pichet, P.: 1996, *NeuroToxicology* **17**(1), 157-168.

Lockhart, W.L., Uthe, J.F., Kenney, A.R., and Mierle, P.M.: 1972, *J. Fish. Res. Bd. Can.* **29**, 1519-1523.

Malm, O., Pfeiffer, W.C., Souza, C.M.M., and Reuther, R.: 1990, *Ambio* **19**, 11-15.

Malm, O., Castro, M.B., Bastos, W.R., Branches, F.P.J., Guimaraes, J.R.D., Zuffo, C.E., and Pfeiffer, W.C.: 1995a, *Sci. Tot al Environ.* **175**, 127-140.

Malm, O., Branches, F.P.J., Akagi H., Castro, M.B., Pfeiffer, W.C., Harada, M., Bastos, W.R., and Kato, H.: 1995b, *Sci. Total Environ.* **175**, 141-150.

Martinelli, L.A., Ferreira, J.R., Forsberg, B.R., and Victor, R.L.: 1988, *Ambio* **17**, 252-254.

Nakanishi, J.: 1992, *Water Report* **2**, 4-5.

Pfeiffer, W.C., Lacerda, L.D., Salomons, W., and Malm, O.: 1993, *Environ. Rev.* **1**, 26-37.

Pfeiffer, W.C., Malm, O., Souza, C.M.M., Lacerda, L.D., Silviera, E.J., and Bastos, W.R.: 1991, *For. Ecol. Manage.* **38**, 239-245.

Plourde, Y., Lucotte M., and Pichet, P.: 1996, *Can. J. Fish. Aquat. Sci.* (*in press*).

Roulet, M., Lucotte, M., Farella, N., Serique, G., Coelho, H., Sousa Passos, C.J., De Jesus da Silva, E., and Scavone de Andrade, P.: 1996a, In: *Proceedings of the Fourth International Conference on Mercury*

as a Global Pollutant, August 4-8, Hamburg, Germany. GKSS-Forschungszentrum Geesthacht, Hamburg, p. 95.
Roulet, M., Lucotte, M., Canuel, R., Rheault, I., Tran, S., De Freitos Gog, Y.G., Farella, N., Souza do Vale R., Sousa Passos, C.J., De Jesus da Silva, E., Mergler, D., Amorim, M.,: 1996b, *Sci. Total Environ. (in press)*.
WHO: 1976, *Environmental Health Criteria 1: Mercury*. World Health Organization, International Program on Chemical Safety, Geneva.
WHO: 1989, *Environmental Health Criteria 86: Mercury-Environmental Aspects*. World Health Organization, International Program on Chemical Safety, Geneva.
WHO: 1990, *Environmental Health Criteria 101: Methylmercury*. World Health Organization, International Program on Chemical Safety, Geneva.

Follow-up of mercury levels in fish, human hair and urine in the Madeira and Tapajós basins, Amazon, Brazil.

MALM, O; GUIMARÃES, JRD; CASTRO, MB; BASTOS, WR; VIANA, JP*; BRANCHES, FJP; SILVEIRA+, EG AND PFEIFFER, WC.

*Instituto de Biofísica CCF°. Univ. Federal do Rio de Janeiro . CCS, Ilha do Fundão, 21949-900. RJ. Brasil. * Univ. of Florida, Gainesville, USA. + Univ. Federal de Rondônia, Porto Velho, RO, Brazil.*

Abstract. Informal economy of gold mining has contaminated some important river basins in Amazon. Follow-up studies on critical compartments showed some areas with high Hg levels in fish as well as in human hair samples. Average Hg in piscivorous fish in the Madeira river itself was 846 ppb (N=284) with a maximum of 3921 ppb. Mercury in fish from non polluted areas in this basin shows high variability, even for single species. A seasonal variation in Hg content was observed, with higher values at the end of the dry season. In the upper Tapajós basin comparable values were found for fish but with a definite decreasing trend downstream. Average value for piscivorous fish in the whole Tapajós basin is 482 ppb (N=122) with a maximum value of 3770 ppb. Hair Hg was higher in fishing villages in the Tapajós (average: 17 ppm; with N=432 and maximum value of 176 ppm) than in the Madeira (average: 9 ppm; N=169; maximum 71 ppm), and data from some areas of the Tapajós suggest a decrease with time. Mercury was much higher in urine of goldshop workers in Santarém (low Tapajós) than in Alta Floresta (high Tapajós) and show a decreasing trend in both cases, probably related to the significant decline in gold mining activities during the study period (1986-1994).

1. Introduction

Non-punctual, mobile, disperse and intermittent sources of mercury (Hg) have released around 2000 metric tons along some main Amazon river basins over the last 20 years. Gold miners use Hg for gold recovery due to some of its very unique properties: capacity of forming amalgams with other metals; high density (as well as gold) so they both tend to concentrate in the heavier sediment fractions; and volatility, allowing the separation of Hg and gold by volatilisation of Hg while burning the amalgam (Pfeiffer & Lacerda, 1988) . This process is very attractive due to its simplicity and low cost, and has been widely used in the Brazilian Amazon basin, in other Latin American countries (Bolivia, Peru, Colombia and Venezuela), as well as in Asia and Africa.

The evolution of total Hg concentrations in fish, human hair and urine was observed in the period 1987-1994 in the Madeira and Tapajós basins to assess environmental and occupational Hg contamination due to gold mining.

Investigations performed during the last 10 years on gold mining areas indicate some aspects of Hg behaviour around emission points as well as along drainages and river basins. The approach used was to look along critical pathways, mainly of methylmercury (MeHg), through piscivorous fauna up to human beings. Occupational exposure to metallic mercury (Hg^0) by inhalation was also evaluated through urine analysis.

2. Material and methods

Different river basins with distinct biogeochemical characteristics were examined. The Madeira river area provided most fish data while human samples were obtained mainly from the Tapajós river basin. Sampling was done in some gold mining areas, riverine communities and cities having strong gold commerce activities. Since man made reservoirs can provide optimum conditions for MeHg formation as well as bioaccumulation, a hydroelectric dam, Samuel reservoir at Madeira river basin was investigated. Some data allowed follow-up studies along the years, such as the Madeira river basin (8 years) or the Tapajós river basin (5 years). Some observations on seasonal variations were made. In the aquatic systems fish were analyzed, since they bioaccumulate and biomagnificate Hg and are a very important item in the diet of local populations. A simplified map of studied areas is presented in Figure 1.

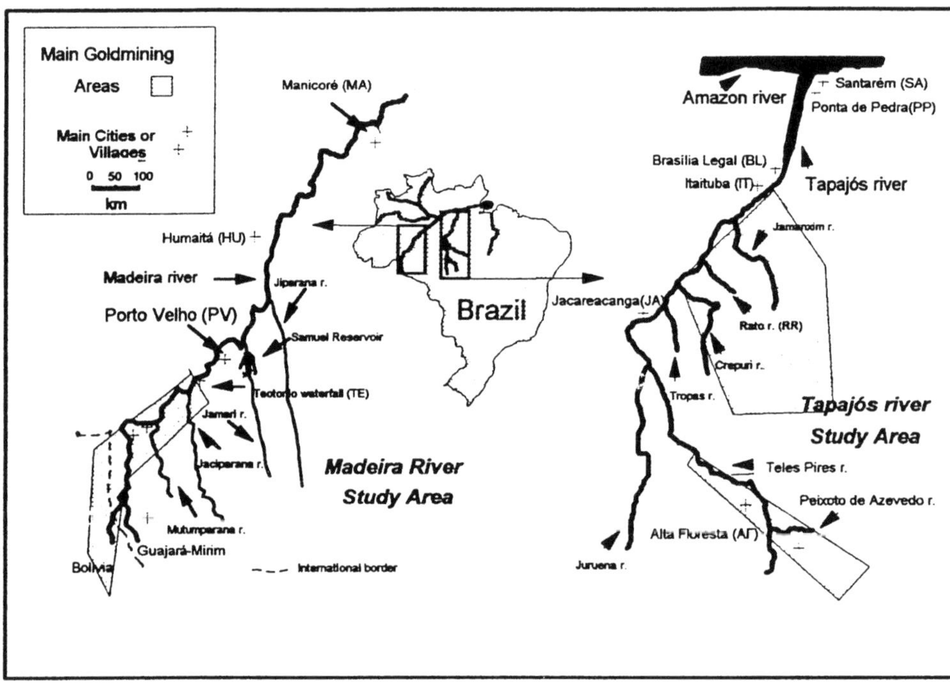

Figure 1. Map of the study areas

Inorganic Hg spread over the environment may be transformed to MeHg, that can then be biomagnified through the food chain. Piscivorous fish from high trophic level are a good indicator for monitoring contaminated rivers and water bodies. Uptake of MeHg through fish ingestion is the main pathway of Hg to humans.

Methylmercury is partly excreted through hair and its concentration is proportional to the blood concentration at the time hair is being formed. We shall discuss fish and hair data from some different riverine cities and villages.

Another situation of high human exposure and toxicity is when metallic Hg is inhaled during the burning of amalgams. This occurs in the gold mining areas as well as in the gold shops. Absorption through the lungs is quite efficient and accumulation occurs in kidneys. Inorganic Hg body burden in humans is better monitored by urine samples.

Analytical techniques for total Hg analysis were developed at the Laboratório de Radioisótopos Eduardo Penna Franca (Malm et al., 1989) and frequently verified through interlaboratory calibration exercises (Malm et al., 1995a; Akagi et al., 1995) as well as with Quality Control programs and analysis of certified reference materials.

Around 1350 samples of fish, human hair and urine were used in this evaluation. This work does not intend to perform a general evaluation of the Hg contamination in an system of such extension and complexity as the Amazon, but rather point out, using our data from two important river basins, the main possibilities and difficulties in identifying trends. The assessment was done here mainly by visual analysis of graphics constructed from these representative data.

3. Results and Discussion

Fish collected at the same places and same time of the year showed a high natural variability in Hg levels that may be explained by the abundant and assorted food offer. A seasonal variability was observed on the same fish species collected at the same location along the year. Rainy season increasing the food offer would probably cause an increase in fat content of fish and consequently a dilution of Hg concentrations, due to fast growth.

The same high diversity in food options for fish could justify the different values observed sometimes inside the same human group. Studies of Hg along hair strands also showed a seasonal variation (Akagi et al., 1994) with the higher values being found during the dry season. This result can reflect the seasonal variation of Hg in fish, but can also be a result of the consumption of different fish species along the year.

Fish is the compartment with the highest number of samples collected. From the Madeira river basin, a total of more than 400 individuals (from around 50 species) were analysed. The very high number of species provides few representative time series from the same species and locations. As expected, a clear pattern is seen with high Hg being observed only in piscivorous species (Figure 2). This group of fish from the Madeira river itself showed a quite high average value (around 850 ppb) reaching values of up to 3,921 ppb. As an example of what is found with several other fish species, *Cichla ocellaris* or "tucunaré" from Samuel reservoir showed no clear relation between Hg concentration and fish weight (Figure 3). This figure also shows an increase in Hg concentration of the fish sampled after an interval of two years (Aug. 1991 - Aug. 1993) at Samuel reservoir, suggesting that Hg levels in fish in this relatively young reservoir is maybe increasing. A seasonal variation was observed on fish collected along the year, as seen in Figures 4 and 5, emphasising the need of comparing only samples collected at the same time of the year.

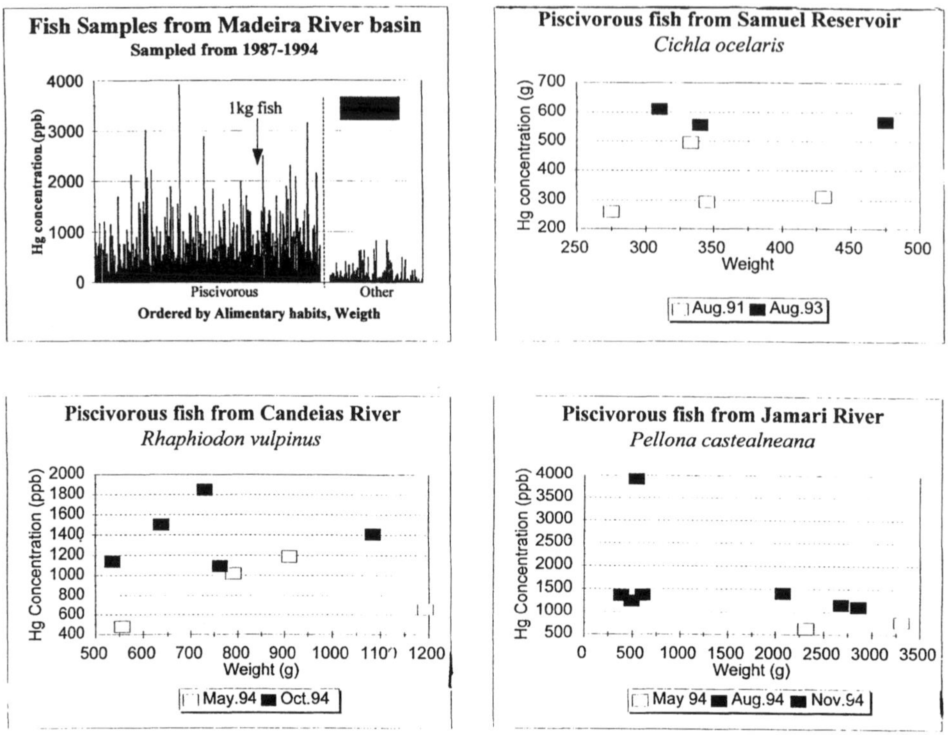

Piscivorous fish collected along the Tapajós river basin present a clear change in Hg concentration depending on sampling sites (Figure 6), showing a decreasing pattern downstream the river basin. This may reflect the influence of several factors, among them the higher Hg discharges in the upper part of the river with lower flow rates. The fish fauna is also quite different along the river. No clear changes between September 1991 and September 1993 were observed for *Cichla ocellaris* (tucunaré) collected at Santarém (Figure 7). There seems to be a weak relationship between total Hg and *C. ocellaris* weight in Santarém, in contrast with the data for the same species in the Madeira river basin, where such relation is not found (Figure 3). Fish collected in Santarém presented in fact such low concentrations that this site could be considered as a control area. Due to the limited number of samples collected at the high reaches of the Tapajós basin, it is difficult to evaluate seasonal variations in Hg concentration, or even identify trends from year to year. Much higher Hg values were observed at the upper part of the Tapajós river at the Teles Pires river close to Alta Floresta city, but fish consumption is low there. In some stretches of those rivers, the kind of fishing activities vary significantly according to the season (Malm et al., 1995b; Lebel et al., 1997).

Hair samples of inhabitants living along the Madeira river showed higher values in the villages of Humaitá and Manicoré, which are both located downstream the main goldmining area and where the population protein diet is more restricted to fish caught locally (Figure 8). Results from hair samples taken at Humaitá three times over four years suggest a decrease in Hg concentration with time, but more follow-up data are necessary to confirm this trend (Figure 9).

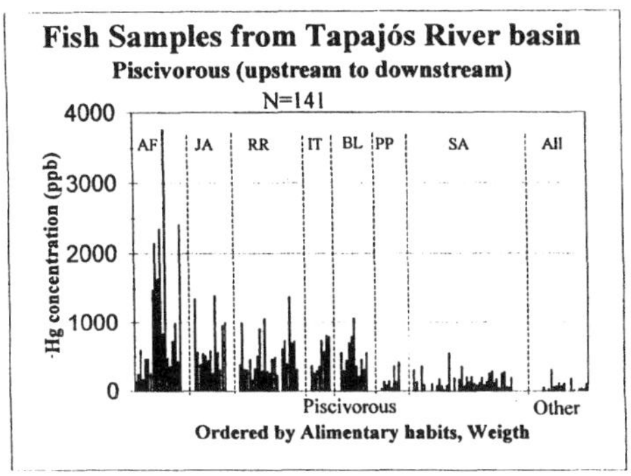

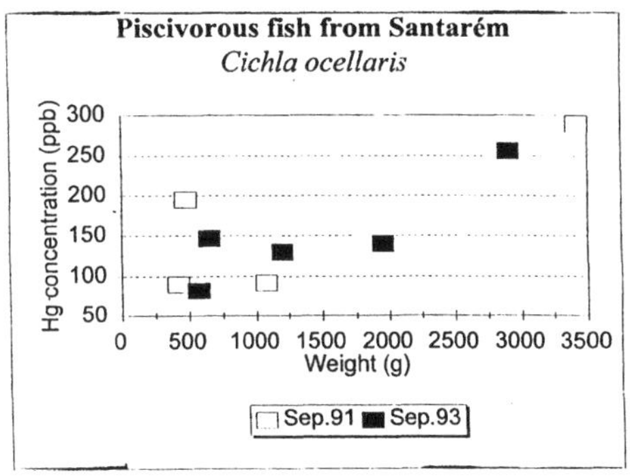

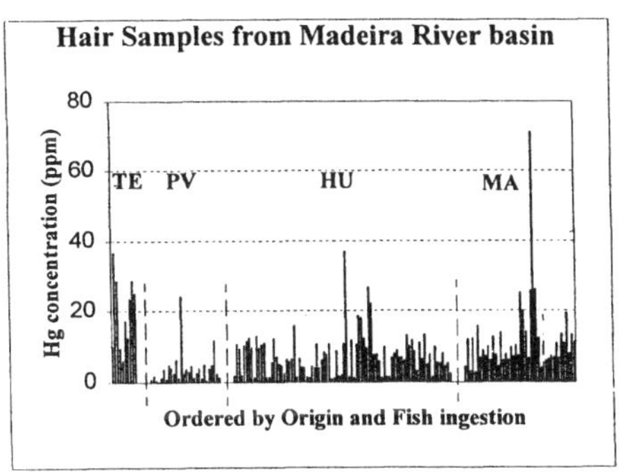

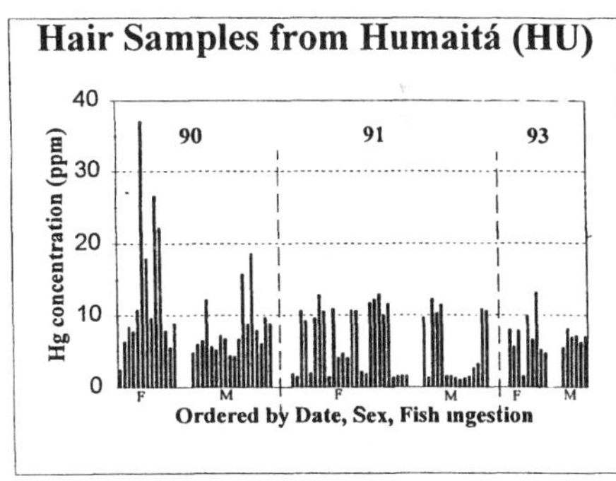

Hair samples from Tapajós river basin individuals (around 430 samples) give better information of Hg on human beings. Hair Hg concentrations from upstream to downstream along the Tapajós river basin (Figure 10) showed trends similar to those found for fish Hg concentrations along the same areas (Figure 6).

Looking at hair Hg of groups of individuals at Brasília Legal, an increase was observed between 1992 and 1993, followed by a decrease in 1994 (Figure 11). If one looks at the results for single individuals along these years, a similar pattern can be identified.

Mercury in urine samples from gold shop workers of two important gold commercial centres showed quite different patterns. At Santarém, very high values were observed in 1991 and 1992 with a sharp decrease in 1994 (Figure 12). Santarém is historically an important gold commercial centre where several gold shops were previously small residences with bad air circulation. This kind of shop predominated during the 80's and early 90's. Today, due to a reduction in gold commerce in the area just a few (and generally big) gold shops remain. In Alta Floresta (Figure 13) the Hg levels in urine were much lower than in Santarém and did not show significant changes between 1991 and 1994. The differences in the Hg levels in urine of gold shop workers between the two cities can be explained by the fact that Alta Floresta is a young city (just 18 years old) and the gold shops there are newer, bigger, and have better ventilation.

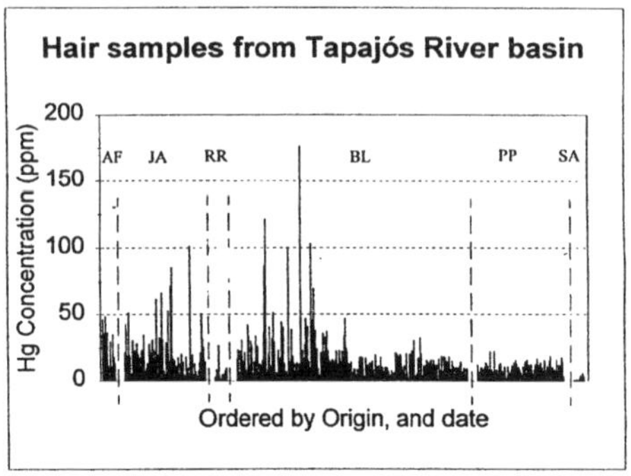

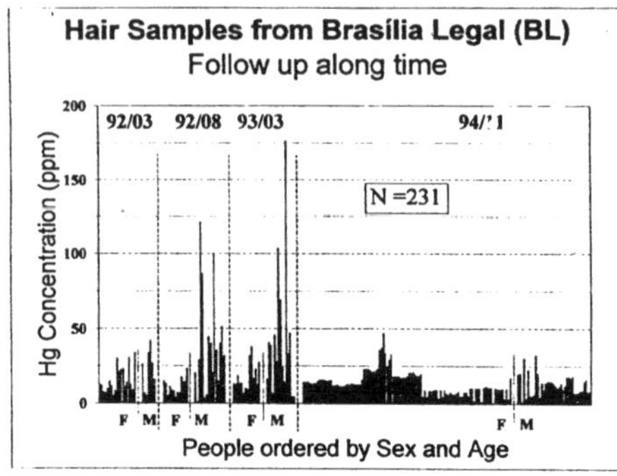

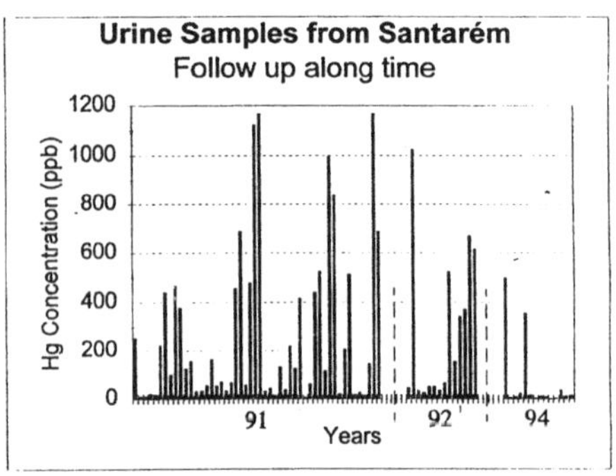

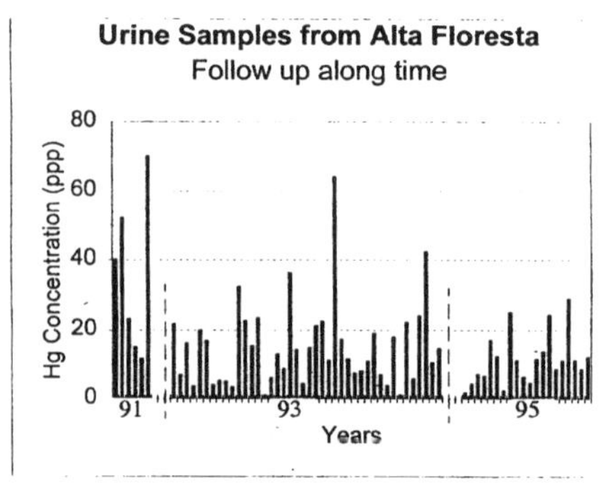

The observed reduction in Hg exposure of the gold shop workers can also be attributed to their increased awareness of the involved risks, as a result of the many in-site investigations made by different research groups. In contrast, in the gold fields (*garimpos*) or in the riverine villages, this alertness is probably lower.

4. Conclusions

- Variability of Hg in fish is quite high, possibly reflecting the high diversity of fish diet and the reduction of food availability to fish during the dry season, the opposite occurring during flooding.

- Riverine populations are critical groups concerning Hg exposure by fish ingestion and must be continuously monitored through hair Hg analysis.
- Due to the high natural variability observed in Hg concentration in some of the compartments studied, more follow up investigations are needed. The extent of such natural variations must be carefully evaluated to help understanding the influence of gold mining.
- Due to seasonal variations, fish and hair samples must be collected at the same time of the year if comparisons are to be made.
- Reduction of Hg levels in hair samples such as the one documented in the medium Tapajós basin can be due to the decrease of Hg concentration in fishes as a consequence of the drastic decline in goldmining activities.
- Reduction of Hg levels in urine samples is more probably also due to this decline rather than to the use of protection or filtration equipments in gold shops.

References

Akagi, H.; Malm, O.;Branches, F.J.P. Kinjo, Y.; Kashima, Y.; Guimarães, J.R.D.; Oliveira, R.B.; Haragushi, K.; Pfeiffer, W.C.; Takizawa, Y. and Kato, H. 1995. Human exposure to Mercury due to goldmining in Tapajós river basin Amazon, Brazil : speciation of mercury in human hair, blood and urine. - Water, Air and Soil Poll. 80:85-94.

Akagi, H.; Kinjo,Y.; Branches, F.; Malm, O.; Harada, M.; Pfeiffer, W.C. and Kato, H. 1994. Methylmercury pollution in Tapajós river basin, Amazon. - Environ. Sciences 3(1), 25 - 32.

Lebel, J; Roulet, M; Mergler, D.; Lucotte, M. and Larribe, F., 1997. Fish diet and mercury exposure in a riparian amazonian population. Water, Air and Soil Pollution, this issue.

Malm, O.; Pfeiffer, W.C.; Bastos, W.R. e Souza, C.M.M. (1989) Utilização do acessório de Geração de Vapor Frio para análise de Hg em investigações ambientais por espectrofotometria de Absorção Atômica. Ciência e Cultura. 41 (1) 88-92.

Malm, O.; Castro, M.B.; Bastos, W.R.; Branches, F.J.P.; Guimarães, J.R.D.; Zuffo, C.E. and Pfeiffer, W.C. 1995a. An assessment of Mercury pollution in different goldmining areas, Amazon Brazil. Science of Total Environment. 175(2) 127-140

Malm, O.; Branches, F.J.P.; Akagi, H.; Castro, M.B.; Pfeiffer, W.C.; Harada, M.; Bastos, W.R. and Kato, H. 1995b Mercury and methylmercury in fish and human hair from Tapajós River Basin, Brazil. Science of Total Environment. 175(2) 141-150.

Pfeiffer, W.C. and Lacerda, L.D. 1988. Mercury imputs into the Amazon region, Brazil. Environ. Technol. Letters,: 9, 325-330.

THE SEYCHELLES CHILD DEVELOPMENT STUDY: RESULTS AND NEW DIRECTIONS THROUGH TWENTY-NINE MONTHS

G. J. MYERS[1], P. W. DAVIDSON[2], C. COX[3], C. F. SHAMLAYE[4], O. CHOISY[4], E. CERNICHIARI[5], A. CHOI[3], J. SLOANE-REEVES[2], C. AXTELL[3], P. GAO[3] and T. W. CLARKSON[5]

[1]Department of Neurology, [2]Department of Pediatrics, [3]Department of Biostatistics, [5]Department of Environmental Medicine, University of Rochester School of Medicine, Rochester, New York . [4]Ministry of Health, The Republic of the Seychelles.

ABSTRACT. The Seychelles Child Development Study was begun in 1986 to prospectively examine the association between child development and prenatal and postnatal methylmercury exposure from a high fish diet. Hair mercury levels from mothers and children are used as the index of exposure. A cross-sectional Pilot Study of 789 infants suggested that prenatal mercury exposure may affect development and that the effect decreased with age independently of exposure. A follow up of 217 Pilot Study children at 66 months of age also suggested that neurodevelopmental effects of prenatal exposure might be present, but the associations were dependent on outcomes in a small number of children. On the basis of the initial results of the Pilot Study a prospective, longitudinal Main Study, with more data on confounding variables and more extensive developmental testing, was begun on a new cohort of 779 children. No association between prenatal exposure and primary neurodevelopmental outcomes was seen at 6 1/2, 19, or 29 months of age. There was an inverse relationship at 29 months in boys only between maternal hair mercury level and activity level, as judged by the examiner during the testing session (one of seven behavioral subscales of the Infant Behavior Record, of the Bayley Scales of Infant Development). In addition to an interaction between maternal hair level and gender, subsequent, secondary analyses are examining interactions between mercury level and a number of socioeconomic factors. Secondary analyses of developmental milestones, similar to those used in the Iraq study, are also under way. Although the association with activity suggests the need for further study of this cohort, no definite adverse neurodevelopmental effects from fetal mercury exposure have been detected through 29 months of age.

In a related study, brains were obtained at autopsy from thirty-two Seychellois infants. Tissue from six different brain regions was examined histologically and analyzed for mercury. No definite histological abnormalities were found. Mercury levels ranged from about 50 ppb to 300 ppb and there was good correlation among brain regions. For 27 brains maternal hair from delivery was available and maternal hair mercury levels correlated well with levels in infant brain.

1. Introduction

This paper provides an updated summary of the results of the Seychelles Child Development Study (SCDS). Marsh *et al.*, (1995) describe the origin of the study, the design, and details on exclusions and confounding variables used in the statistical analysis. Shamlaye *et al.*, (1995) present the background of the study, including information on the Republic of Seychelles and demographic data on the pilot and main cohorts.

The analytical and dosimetry aspects of the study are presented by Cernichiari *et al.*, (1995a). This includes the methods for collection, transport, and analysis of maternal and child hair samples. These are used as the main biological monitoring medium for pre and postnatal methylmercury exposure. Sampling of blood, breast milk and fish is also described, as well as the collection of blood samples for measurement of lead and PCBs.

Clinical and epidemiological data have been presented in a series of papers. The cross-sectional pilot study was described and results of the primary evaluation of the cohort discussed by Myers *et al.*, (1995a). This was followed by a report on a subset of the pilot cohort examined at 66 months of age (Myers *et al.*, 1995b). Enrollment of the Main Study cohort was described and evaluations at 6 1/2 months of age discussed by Myers *et al.*, (1995c). Testing procedures and the resulting distributions were described in Davidson *et al.*, (1995a). This was followed by a description of the results of the 19 and 29-month evaluations of the main cohort (Davidson *et al.*, 1995b). Subsequently, secondary analyses have been undertaken. The first of these is examining the associations between maternal hair levels and developmental milestones similar to those used in studies in Iraq. The second is examining interactive effects between prenatal exposure and various socioeconomic factors, including maternal intelligence, family income and the home environment.

In a related but separate study, a series of thirty-two brains was obtained at autopsy from infants dying from a variety of causes. After fixation in formalin, histopathological examinations and mercury analyses were performed on 6 brain regions (Lapham *et al.*, 1995). For a subset of 27 brains, samples of maternal and infant blood and maternal hair were also available for mercury analysis. This allowed correlation of mercury levels from biological monitoring media (maternal hair and blood) with levels in the target organ (infant brain) (Cernichiari *et al.*, 1995b).

Statistical analyses for both clinical studies included multiple logistic or linear regression using all covariates (full model) as well as only those covariates felt to be most important in Seychelles (reduced model). For each analysis an interaction between gender and mercury exposure was also examined.

2. Results

2.1 PILOT STUDY

In this cross-sectional study, 789 Seychellois infants and toddlers were enrolled and examined at ages between one and 25 months (Myers *et al.*, 1995a). This examination included a medical history and complete neurological evaluation, as well as administration of the Denver Developmental Screening Test - Revised (DDST). Based on results from studies in Iraq, two neurological outcomes were selected as primary endpoints in addition to the overall examination. These were muscle tone and deep tendon reflexes.

Table 1 summarizes the results of the statistical analysis of the primary endpoints from the pilot study. An association between maternal hair levels and scores on the DDST was found. Separate effects of gender and age at testing were also found. This result was present only when scores of *abnormal* were combined with *questionable* scores, and disappeared when the analysis combined *questionable* scores with *normal.* The standard scoring for the DDST is to treat only abnormal scores as failures. No

TABLE I

Regression Analysis from the Primary Analysis Plan for the Pilot Study. Results of Significance Tests (p-values)+

Examinations	Test for Interaction		Test for Regression Model				Mercury Effect	
			With Interaction		Without Interaction			
	Full	Reduced	Full	Reduced	Full	Reduced	Full	Reduced
First exam								
DDST-R*	0.41	0.43	--	--	0.21	0.04	0.044**	0.031**
Overall Neurological	0.15	0.10	--	--	<0.0001	<0.0001	0.13	0.16
Muscle tone	0.91	0.76	--	--	<0.0001	<0.0001	0.19	0.20
Deep Tendon Reflexes	0.78	0.63	--	--	0.056	0.02	0.58	0.61

+From Myers et al., 1995d
* DDST-R: Denver Developmental Screening Test-Revised
**One-sided

association between the results of the neurological examination and maternal hair level was found.

In preparation for the main study evaluation, a subset of 217 of these children was re-examined at 66 months of age (Myers *et al.*, 1995b). This involved a comprehensive examination, including tests of intelligence and achievement. A total of nine different endpoints was analyzed, using multiple regression models similar to those used in other phases of the Pilot Study. A significant association was found between maternal hair levels and global intellectual function, perceptual ability, and language function (auditory comprehension and total language). When a small number (three or four depending on the particular endpoint) of outliers and influential scores were removed, this effect disappeared for every endpoint except auditory comprehension. (Receptive Language). As an illustration of the effects of outliers and influential points, consider the analyses for the McCarthy GCI, a test of global intellectual function. Figure 1 shows a plot of GCI scores, adjusted for covariates vs. maternal hair levels. Because the test scores have been adjusted, the slope of the regression line is the regression coefficient for mercury in the full regression model. The three outliers for this analysis can be clearly seen in this plot. All three scores were less than 60, several standard deviations below the average score for the entire group. The maternal hair levels for these outliers range from less than 5 to 23, the second largest in the data set. The latter point had a highly influential effect on the regression coefficient for mercury. The final interpretation of these results must await the analysis of the 5.5 year tests from the Main Study.

2.2 MAIN STUDY

Following the initial phase of the pilot study, a prospective, longitudinal study with a new cohort was begun with testing at ages of 6 1/2, 19, 29 and 66 months. The endpoints and covariates were expanded on the basis of results from the pilot study and an examination setting conducive to test administration was established (Marsh *et al.*,

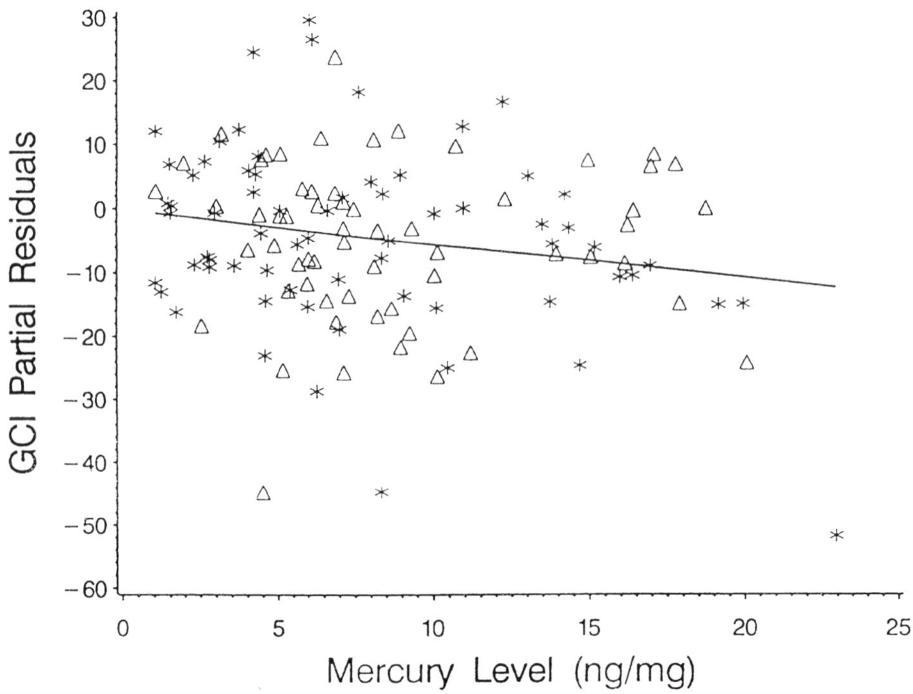

Fig 1. A plot of the partial residuals for mercury from the regression analysis of the GCI scores. Males (Δ) and females (*) are labeled separately. The partial residual represents the GCI score adjusted for all the other variables in the regression except mercury. The partial residual is calculated by combining the residual from the original regression with the mercury effect. The straight line in the figure is the regression line for the partial residuals on the maternal hair levels. The slope of this line is the regression coefficient for mercury in the original multiple regression analysis. (From Myers et al., 1995b).

1995; Myers *et al.* , 1995c). The 6 1/2 month examination included the same outcomes as the pilot study (neurological examination and DDST). In addition, the Fagan Infantest was used to measure visual recognition memory as well as visual attention. Outcomes from testing at 19 and 29 months of age were taken from the Bayley Scales of Infant Development (BSID). These included the Mental (MDI) and Psychomotor (PDI) Development Indices, and the Infant Behavior Record (IBR) at 29 months. The list of covariates was enlarged to provide more information on socioeconomic factors, including administration of the Caldwell-Bradley Home Observation for measurement of the child's environment.

The results of the statistical analyses for main study at enrollment (6 1/2 months of age) are summarized in Table 2. No association between maternal hair levels and the DDST-R, the endpoints from the neurological examination, the Fagan test of visual recognition memory, or the attention subscore from the Fagan test was found (Myers *et al.*, 1995c).

At 19 and 29 months of age, no association between maternal hair levels and the BSID, MDI or PDI was found (Davidson *et al.*, 1995a). However, on the more subjective behavioral subscales of the IBR, one of the seven measures, activity, did

TABLE II

Regression Analysis from the Primary Analysis for the Main Study. Results of Significance Tests (p values)*

Examination	Tests for Interaction		Test for Regression Model				Mercury Effect	
			With Interaction		Without Interaction			
	Full	Reduced	Full	Reduced	Full	Reduced	Full	Reduced
Six month exam								
Overall neurological	--	--	--	--	--	--	--	--
Muscle Tone	0.58	0.40	--	--	0.0003	0.0004	0.92	0.85
Deep tendon reflexes	0.07	0.18	--	--	0.59	0.49	0.40	0.26
Fagan Scale	0.20	0.20	--	--	0.46	0.14	0.74	0.56
Attention scale	0.99		--	--	0.08	0.03	0.25	0.48
19 month exam								
BSID-MDI	0.53	0.44	--	--	<0.0001	<0.0001	0.12	0.32
BSID-PDI	0.49	0.61	--	--	0.09	0.05	0.21	0.47
BSID-Kohen-Raz	0.87	0.33	--	--	0.11	0.27	0.76	0.91
29 month exam								
BSID-MDI	0.63	0.58	--	--	<0.0001	<0.0001	0.08	0.23
BSID-PDI	0.11	0.74	--	--	0.32	0.67	0.79	0.95
BSID-IBR Activity	0.047	0.0075	<0.0001	<0.0001	--	--	0.033(M) 0.52(F)	0.0004(M) 0.87(F)
BSID-IBR Exam rating	0.66	0.64	--	--	<0.0001	<0.0001	0.64	0.27
BSID-IBR mother	0.33	0.30	--	--	<0.0001	<0.0001	0.76	0.73
BSID-IBR coop.	0.35	0.48	--	--	<0.0001	<0.0001	0.35	0.59
BSID-IBR attention	0.26	0.34	--	--	0.04	0.03	0.44	0.29

BSID: Bayley Scales of Infant Development; MDI: Mental Development Index; PDI: Physical Development
Index; IBR: Infant Behavioral Rating
*From Myers et al., 1995d

show an association with mercury exposure. The relationship was present only in males, and predicted lower activity with increasing maternal hair levels (Davidson *et al.*, 1995b).

Following the analysis of data on the primary endpoints from the first three examinations, secondary outcomes are also being examined for an effect of prenatal exposure. Since the outcomes in the Iraq study were based on developmental milestones, similar endpoints were also defined for the Main Study cohort. These are ages of walking (walking without support) and talking (saying words other than *mama* or *dada*). Data on these milestones were obtained as part of the 19 month evaluation. In Iraq an abnormal motor response was defined as not walking by 18 months; in the Main Study cohort, only three children did not walk by 18 months of age. For these analyses the actual ages of achievement of the milestones will be used. The same regression models will be used as for analysis of the primary endpoints.

Following Schroeder *et al.* (1985) an additional series of secondary analyses are examining differential effects of prenatal exposure according to levels of various socioeconomic factors. Specifically, two different regression models were developed; the first included interactions between prenatal exposure and the following socioeconomic factors: birth weight, home environment, maternal age, maternal intelligence, parental education, duration of breast feeding, and monthly income. The second model included all these interactions and in addition interactions between gender and the socioeconomic factors. Analyses are being performed using both of these models for the primary endpoints from the first three examinations.

2.3 NEUROPATHOLOGICAL STUDIES

While the clinical studies were underway, plans were made to obtain brains from autopsies of infants (Lapham *et al.*, 1995). Brains from 32 infants were obtained. Causes of death varied, but none directly involved the central nervous system. Six areas of the brain (frontal cortex, occipital cortex, temporal cortex with hippocampus, basal ganglia with thalamus, cerebellum, and pons with medulla) were examined histologically and analyzed for mercury after fixation in formalin. Levels of mercury ranged from ≤50 ppb to >300 ppb. Levels of mercury in each brain region correlated well with levels in other regions. No differences in mercury levels were observed between gray and white matter.

Histological examination of the six brain areas revealed no definite neuropathological abnormalities (Lapham *et al.*, 1995), although some brains exhibited low-grade, non-specific changes. Variable numbers of reactive plump astrocytes were present in the white matter of 22 brains, and increased numbers of reactive microglia were also seen in the white matter in 24 brains. However, no association was found between the severity of these effects and levels of mercury in the brains.

In a subset of 27 brains, maternal hair and blood mercury levels at delivery as well as blood mercury levels in the infants at autopsy were available. Significant correlations were found between levels of mercury in all these media (Cernichiari *et al.*, 1995b). These are shown schematically in Figure 2. The six correlations between maternal hair levels and six different regions of infant brain were between 0.60 and 0.80, with other correlations as indicated. The p-values for all of these correlations were less than 0.01. The figure also shows an indirect comparison between maternal hair and infant brain by comparison with levels in maternal and infant blood. Both the direct and the indirect comparisons indicate a high degree of association between maternal hair and infant brain. This shows that maternal hair mercury levels during pregnancy can serve as an accurate and reliable biological monitor for mercury levels in the developing brain.

3. Discussion

The Seychelles Pilot Study found a relationship between fetal mercury exposure and neurodevelopment at enrollment and a suggestion of an effect in a subgroup at the 66-month evaluation. However, this latter association was highly dependent on a small number of outliers and influential scores. It is still uncertain whether an association exists between fetal mercury exposure at levels found naturally in ocean fish and neurodevelopment. Although both outliers and influential points are to be expected in the kinds of regression analyses which are required in this study, the presence of

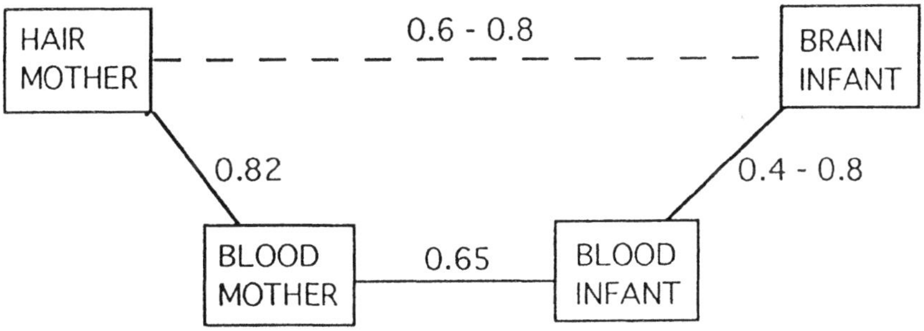

Fig. 2. Direct and indirect routes of comparison of mercury levels in maternal hair and infant brain. The number adjacent to the lines are correlation coefficients. (From Cernichiari et al., 1995b)

statistical outliers and influential points complicates both the analysis and the interpretation of the results. The definition of an outlier which we used is a purely statistical one; a test score is an outlier if the residual (the difference between the actual score and the value predicted by the regression model using information on all of the predictor variables) is large as judged by the goodness of fit of the model. Assuming that the model is correct, it is possible to standardize the residuals using estimates of variability from the model, to behave approximately like normal deviates (Z scores). On this scale a (Z) value of greater than 3 or less than -3 is unusually large. Such points are inconsistent with the remainder of the data and should be removed for final analysis.

Outliers may or may not represent unusually high or low scores on a given test. This is because being an outlier depends both on the actual test score and on the pattern of predictor variables. (A specific score which is an outlier for one child may not be an outlier for a child with a different pattern of variables.) Once a point has been identified as an outlier it is important to check all of the data for this observation. This is necessary both to check for errors and to determine if the child may be developmentally delayed. In the case of Seychelles, outliers were typically unusually low scores. For the 66 month pilot study for example, the outliers were all low scores, and upon review of both the data base and pediatric records a number of developmental delays were identified. It was also noted that maternal hair levels for these outliers included both low and relatively high values. From a statistical point of view it is reasonable to drop outliers from the main analysis since these are inconsistent with the results of the regression model. Conclusions from the statistical analysis should be representative of the whole group, not a few individuals.

From a clinical point of view, one may want to ask whether the potential effects represented by a small number of test scores, which are identified as statistical outliers could possibly be due to prenatal exposure. This question raises a number of issues. The first is whether such severe effects have ever been seen in a population of exposure levels such as this, and what factors might explain the difference between this small number of individuals and the remainder of the cohort. This is related to the adequacy of the regression model; it is always possible that an important covariate has not been identified which would change the results of the analysis considerably. It must also be kept in mind that the Seychelles study was not designed to look for severe effects in a very small number of children. Rather the opposite is true; we hypothesized a dose-effect relationship in the entire population. Data collection procedures and statistical analyses were designed with this hypothesis in mind, and additional data may be required to address the question of severe effects in a small number of children.

Testing limitations may also temper interpretation of our results. None of the developmental tests had been extensively used in Seychelles before the study began. We may not have the kind of normative data which might be helpful in interpreting extreme test scores. In any case conclusions should clearly be based on the analysis with outliers removed, both for scientific and statistical reasons. The results of the analysis must, however, be interpreted with these issues in mind.

The question of influential points is somewhat less complicated, if only because these points are not actually removed for the final analysis. An influential point is one which has a relatively large effect on the results of the statistical analysis, without necessarily being an outlier. Since our study focused on the effects of prenatal exposure, we limited the question of influence to the effect of the maternal hair level. Thus we ignored the question of influence with regard to the covariates. For the maternal hair level effect the influential points are primarily those with relatively large maternal hair levels; the distribution is fairly skewed and a small number of such values is to be expected. These points may be influential almost entirely because we do not have more values in this upper range. Therefore we remove points which have been identified as influential, in order to assess the extent to which the results depend on these individual values. If the results change considerably when a small number of influential points is removed, then an additional degree of caution must be added to the interpretation. We may simply not have enough data in the region where effects begin to appear.

The assessment of influence is based on the standardized change in the regression coefficient for maternal hair level when a particular point is removed. A limitation of this approach is that points are examined individually. Although this procedure has proven to be useful in identifying influential points, it may be that the situation is different if more than one point is removed. It is not difficult to make up examples in which a given point is or is not influential by itself, and the opposite is true when a second point is also removed. The whole question of influence is highly multidimensional, and is another consequence of variables we cannot control in an observational study.

The Seychelles Child Development Study has found a high correlation between maternal hair mercury levels at delivery and neonatal brain levels, confirming the value of maternal hair as a biological marker for fetal exposure to methylmercury. No consistent neurodevelopmental effects of prenatal exposure have been found through 29 months of age.

Acknowedgments

This research was supported by grants ES-01247, T32 ES07271, and ES-05497 from the National Institutes of Health (NIH) by a grant from the Food and Drug Administration, USDHHS, and by the Ministry of Health, Republic of the Seychelles and the Government of Sweden.

This study was conducted with the collaboration of the Seychelles Child Development group described below.

The Seychelles Child Development Study Group

Analytical. T. Clarkson, E. Cernichiari, M. Langdon (Tech). *Biostatistics.* C. Cox (Chief), M. Tanner (Biostatistician), A. Choi (Analyst-Programmer), P. Gao (Biostatistician), C. Axtell (Biostatistician), Y. Wang (Biostatistician); *Clinical:*: University of Rochester School of Medicine and Dentistry, Rochester, NY: G. Myers (Chief), D. Marsh (Chief, 1985-1990), P. Davidson (Psychological Testing), J. Sloane-Reeves (Tech.). Ministry of Health, Republic of Seychelles: O. Choisy (Coordinator), J. Etienne (Project Nurse), M.A. Payet (Project Nurse), Sr. Claire Hoareau (Maternity Superintendent); *Data Coordination.* University of Rochester: G. Myers (Chief), E. Cernichiari (Coordinator), E. Forsythe (Data Control Clerk): *Epidemiology*: C. Shamlaye. *Pathology/Morphology*: R. Baggs, R. Brewer, L. Lapham.

References

Cernichiari, E., Brewer, R., Myers, G. J., *et al.*: 1995b, *NeuroToxicology*, 16(4),705-709.
Cernichiari, E., Toribara, T. Y., Liang, L., *et al.*: 1995a, *Neurotoxicology* , 16(4),613-628.
Davidson, P.W., Myers, G. J., Cox, C., *et al.*: 1995, *Neurotoxicology,* 16(4), 665-676.
Davidson, P.W., Myers, G. J., Cox, C., *et al.*: 1995b, *NeuroToxicology,* 16(4):677-688.
Lapham, L.W., Cernichiari, E., Cox ,C., *et al.*: 1995, *Neurotoxicology*, 16(4):689-703.
Marsh, D.O., Clarkson, T.W., Myers, G. J., et al.: 1995, *Neurotoxicology* , 16(4), 583-596.
Myers, G. J., Davidson, P.W., Cox, C., *et al.*: 1995b, *Neurotoxicology* , 16(4), 639-652.
Myers, G. J., Davidson, P.W., Cox, C., *et al.*: 1995d, *Neurotoxicology*,16(4), 711-716..
Myers, G. J., Marsh, D.O., Cox ,C., *et al.*: 1995a, *Neurotoxicology* , 16(4), 629-638.
Myers, G. J., Marsh, D.O., Davidson, P.W., et al.: 1995c, *Neurotoxicology* , 16(4), 653-664.
Schroeder, S., Hawk, B., Ottow, D., et al.: 1985, *Environ. Res*. 38, 144-154.
Shamlaye, C.F., Marsh, D.O., Myers, G. J., et al.: 1995, *Neurotoxicology* , 16(4),598-612.

EXPOSURE PATTERNS AND LONG TERM SEQUELAE ON ADULTS AND CHILDREN IN TWO CANADIAN INDIGENOUS COMMUNITIES EXPOSED TO METHYLMERCURY.

BRIAN WHEATLEY[1], SYLVAIN PARADIS[1], MARYSE LASSONDE[2], MARIE-FRANCE GIGUERE[1] and SERGE TANGUAY[1].

[1]*Research and Development, Environmental Contaminants, Medical Services Branch, Health Canada, Room 1150, Jeanne-Mance Building, Tunney's Pasture, Ottawa, Ontario, K1A 0L3, Canada;*
[2] *Départment de Psychologie, C.P. 6128, Université de Montréal, Succ. Centre Ville, Montréal, Québec, H4A 2X9*

Abstract Health Canada has been collecting data on Inuit and First Nations' methylmercury (MeHg) levels for 25 years. A national overview has been completed and more focussed analyses have now been initiated. This paper deals with two interdependent analytical components: 1) a longitudinal overview of the two most extensively sampled communities in Canada: Grassy Narrows and Whitedog, the residents of which were exposed to 'point source' mercury pollution in the 1970's; 2) fetal and post-natal exposure to mercury in these two communities including an outline of the First Nation MeHg child development pilot project in the two communities. A retrospective analysis of Grassy Narrows and Whitedog shows a decreasing MeHg trend in both communities. In Grassy Narrows the average individual annual peak methylmercury level in blood has decreased significantly, from 23.80 ppb (range 1.50-322.90) in 1976 to 7.5 ppb (1.7-46.7) in 1995 ($r=-0.65$, $p<0.001$). In Whitedog the average peak has also decreased significantly, from 12.87 ppb (1.50-172.00) in 1976 to 6.1 ppb (1.7-33.3) in 1995 ($r=-0.59$, $p<0.005$). However, behind these positive trends is the reality of two communities still suffering the effects of disrupted lifestyles and socio-cultural damage. A number of cord blood samples, maternal blood samples, and samples from women of child-bearing age from these communities have been in the "risk" group (according to the 1990 WHO guidelines). We are therefore now assessing the long term effects of fetal exposure in the communities. Standard clinical examinations in the past failed to prove abnormalities attributable to methylmercury but did not include subtle neuropsychological development tests. Many of the fetally exposed children are now in secondary school. Therefore, we have initiated a pilot project to assess long term effects of methylmercury exposure on the neuropsychological development of these children whose fetal exposure we know. The pilot child development project which was initiated in 1995 in Grassy Narrows and Whitedog, with community support, includes four main components: i) a school records review, looking at attendance, marks, and atypical behaviour; ii) teachers' questionnaires, targeting child behaviour; iii) an in-depth neuropsychological test battery focussing on subtle factors, such as memory, attention, executive functions, perceptual functions and sensory / motor development; and iv) hair sampling, providing current MeHg levels to correlate with results from the previous sampling and findings from the first three components. An overview of progress is given.

1. Introduction

In the 1960s and early 1970s mercury was discharged from a chlor-alkali plant into the English-Wabigoon river system in northern Ontario (Rudd *et al.*, 1983). Down stream of the plant were two native communities: Grassy Narrows and Whitedog. These communities depended heavily on fish from the river system both for subsistence food and as an economic base from guiding sport fishermen. The mercury, having been methylated in the aquatic ecosystem, was bio-accumulated in fish to levels up to 24 ppm (Bishop and Neary, 1976). This resulted in exposure of the residents of Grassy Narrows and Whitedog, who were eating the fish, to high levels of methylmercury (MeHg). The highest human level seen was in one individual who attained 660 ppb in blood in 1971. The program developed by Health Canada in response to this crisis was later expanded to cover the majority of native communities in Canada and is reported elsewhere (Wheatley and Paradis, 1995;

1996). This paper concentrates on the communities of Grassy Narrows and Whitedog. It will describe the changing pattern of exposure of residents of these communities over the past twenty years. It will also outline the initial steps which have been taken to address fetal and post-natal exposure to mercury, based on known cord blood levels, current hair levels and current neuropsychological testing of the children.

2. Methodology/Findings

With the exception of the cord blood samples, the majority of the samples analysed were hair (Wheatley, 1979). Hair is the best biological indicator of human MeHg exposure, providing temporal information when analysis is carried out on sequential 1 cm samples (WHO, 1976). However, for historical reasons, within the program, results have always been reported as ppb in blood (Wheatley and Paradis, 1995). Based on research with Canadian First Nations, a factor of 1:300 was used to convert from hair levels to blood levels (Phelps *et al.,* 1980). Over the past 20 years, the number of centimeters tested has increased on average from 4 per 12 cm hair sample in 1975-79 to 6 for the period of 1995-96. The number of centimeters tested could have been larger but analyses were performed every second centimeter to cover the largest temporal span possible up to 12 cms. For each hair sample the level reported, for risk assessment purposes, has always been the maximum level in any one sample. In 1975, as part of risk assessment, the sampling strategy was to target heavy fish eaters and heads of households, as representatives of household exposure, with follow up testing of family members as appropriate. In 1995 the strategy was to obtain hair samples from those with previous high MeHg levels. However, during both periods, any individuals who were concerned about their mercury levels were sampled if the request was made by the individual. All samples were analyzed by the same central laboratory using the same methodology throughout the program (Farant *et al.,* 1981). The laboratory is currently running the international hair mercury QA/QC program.

Community	Sampling year	Mean	Minimum	Maximum	# of individuals	Population
Grassy Narrows	1976	23.8	1.5	322.9	239	421
	1995	7.5	1.7	46.7	116	597
Whitedog	1976	12.9	1.5	172.0	292	555
	1995	6.1	1.7	33.3	52	774

Table I. Grassy Narrows and Whitedog: Range of Maximum MeHg levels (ppb) for individuals in 1976 and 1995

A retrospective analysis of results (community, cohort and individual) from Grassy Narrows and Whitedog between 1976 and 1995 shows a downward trend in methylmercury levels in both communities (Table I). Although the two communities have similar trends, they vary in the ranges of MeHg levels and the magnitude of the changes. For this reason, we have decided to present concurrently the results and graphs of the analytical results. Using a Pearson correlation of community average MeHg level over the past 20 years, a significant decreasing trend has been identified in Grassy Narrows ($r = -0.65$, $p<0.001$) from an average of 23.80 ppb (individual range: 1.50 to 322.90 ppb) in 1976 to 7.46 ppb (range: 1.67 to 46.67 ppb) in 1995. The same decreasing trend was observed in Whitedog ($r = -0.59$, $p<0.005$) from an average of 12.87 ppb (range: 1.50 to 172.00 ppb) in 1976 to 6.08 ppb (range: 1.67 to 33.33 ppb) in 1995.

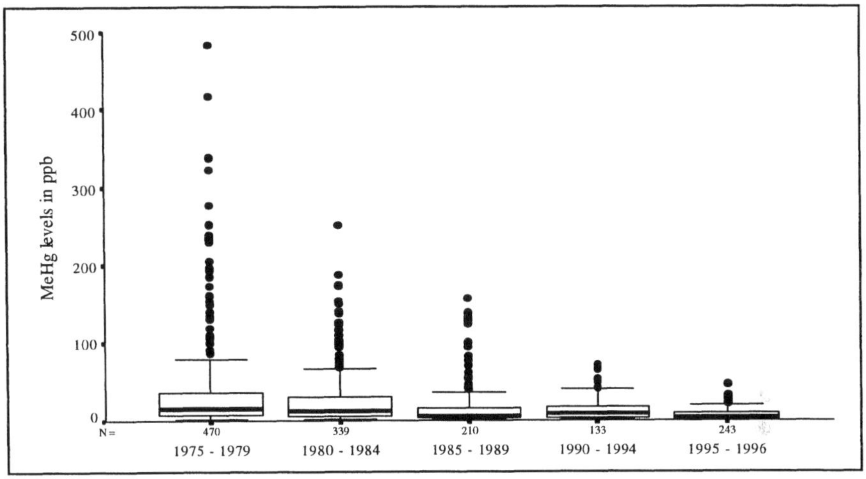

Fig. 1 Grassy Narrows: Box Plot of Maximum MeHg levels from 1975 to 1996 for each individual in each period

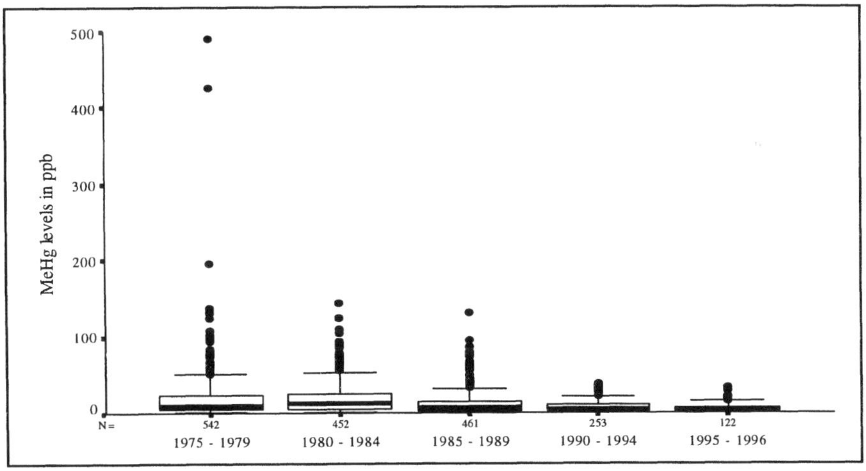

Fig. 2 Whitedog: Box Plot of Maximum MeHg levels from 1975 to 1996 for each individual in each period

From the box plots of results from Grassy Narrows and Whitedog showing maximum levels in each test in five time intervals (Figures 1 and 2), the decrease in the MeHg levels is very evident. However, the proportion of outliers has stayed approximately the same over each period although in the 1990-1994 and 1995-1996 samples all are less than 100 ppb. The median MeHg levels have decreased, as has the overall distribution, especially since 1990.

Community	Maximum MeHg levels in ppb	1975-1980 Percentage of individuals	1995-1996 Percentage of individuals
Grassy Narrows	< 20	21.4	79.6
(N = 103)	≥ 20 and < 100	60.2	20.4
	≥ 100	18.4	
Whitedog	< 20	59.4	93.7
(N = 32)	≥ 20 and < 100	37.5	6.3
	≥ 100	3.1	

Table II Mean annual individual maximum in each period for the same individuals

To ensure consistency of the findings we also reviewed a cohort of individuals in each community where the results from these same individuals in 1975-1980 and 1995-1996 are known (Table II). Points of interest in this table include: i) for the 1995-96 period, there are no results above 100 ppb; ii) for this same period for each community most of the levels are below 20 ppb; and iii) the proportion in the 20-100 ppb group has reduced from 60.2% (Grassy Narrows) and 37.5% (Whitedog) to 20.4% and 6.3% over the 20 year period. Considering both communities together, this decreasing trend is significant (paired t-test, $t = 8.21$, $df = 134$, $p<0.001$). The average MeHg level for 1975-80 was 56.08 ppb (sd = 68.74) compared to 10.59 ppb (sd = 9.5) in 1995-96. Only 4 individuals showed an increase in MeHg levels compared to 128 who decreased, while 3 maintained the same levels. The decreasing trend in MeHg levels was also significant for both Grassy Narrows ($t = 7.83$, $df = 102$, $p<0.001$) and Whitedog ($t = 3.95$, $df = 31$, $p<0.001$) when the 2 communities were evaluated separately.

Figure 3 directly compares individual levels from 1975-80 with levels from 1995-96. All individuals with previously high levels are now much lower. In this figure, both communities have been included. In addition to the dramatic individual changes, attention should be focussed on the scales of the axes. While the Y scale (1975 to 1980) ranges from 0 to 500 ppb, the X scale (1995-1996) range is from 0 to 50 ppb. The magnitude has therefore decreased significantly, roughly by a factor of 10.

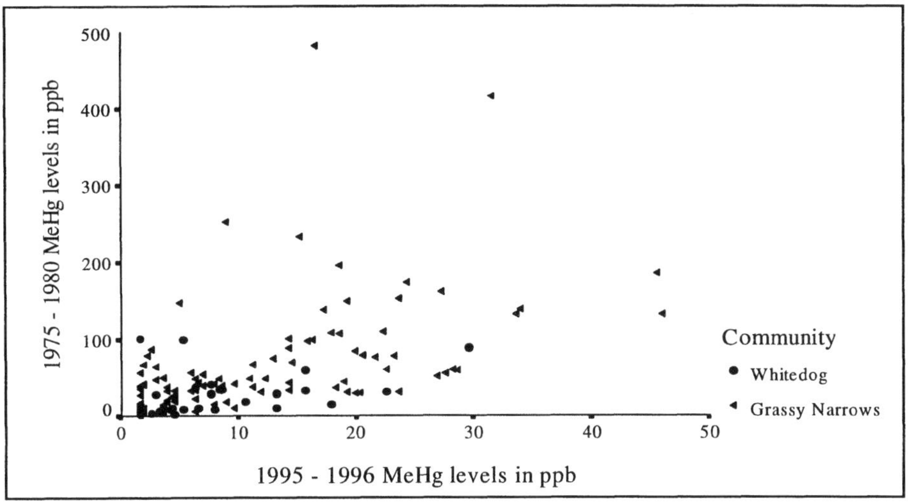

Fig. 3 Grassy Narrows and Whitedog: Comparison of maximum individual 1995-1996 MeHg levels and 1975-1980 levels for the same individuals

Also, at the individual level, the composite series of results from a fishing guide from Grassy Narrows (Wheatley & Paradis, 1995), which we have now extended to 1995, confirms a falling trend (Figure 4).

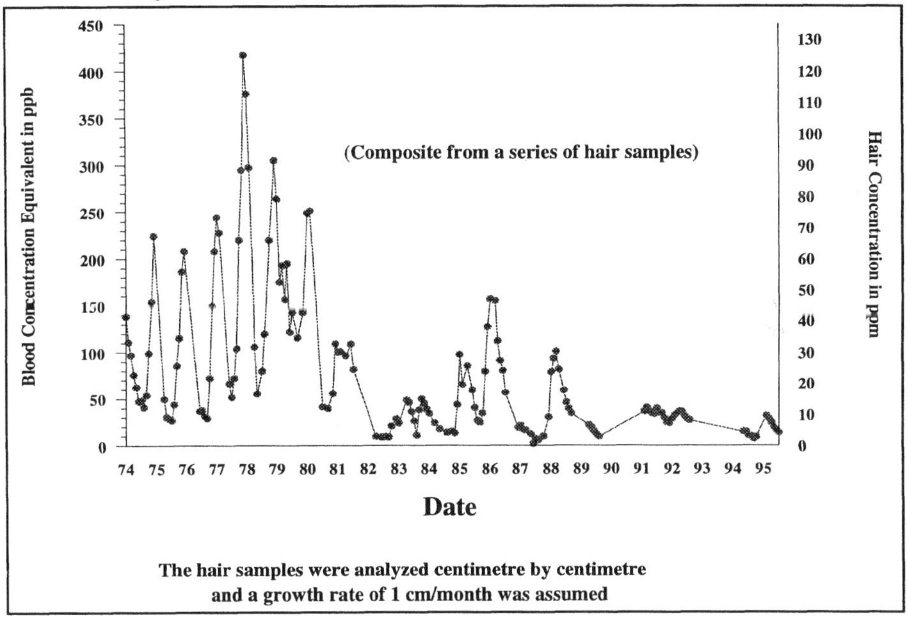

Fig. 4 Seasonal variation of mercury level in a fishing guide from Grassy Narrows Reserve, Ontario

However, behind these positive trends is the reality of two communities still suffering the effects of disrupted lifestyles and socio-cultural damage, contributed to by the loss of their subsistence food and economic base due to methylmercury in the aquatic ecosystem (Shkilnyk, 1985; Erikson, 1994; Wheatley, M.A., 1996).

Community	Sample type	Total number of individuals	# of individuals ≥ 30 ppb	Percent ≥ 30 ppb
Grassy Narrows	Cord Blood (1978-1987)	156	4	2.6
	Maternal Blood (1978-1981)	44	6	13.6
	Child bearing age women (1975-1995)	155	38	24.5
Whitedog	Cord Blood (1978-1987)	153	13	8.5
	Maternal Blood (1978-1981)	42	5	11.9
	Child bearing age women (1975-1995)	230	37	16.1

Table III Grassy Narrows and Whitedog MeHg levels above or equal to 30 ppb

Part of our review of the current situation in Grassy Narrows and Whitedog included recognition of current international concern regarding the effects of fetal and neonatal exposure. We knew that a number of cord blood samples taken from the communities in the past, as well as maternal blood samples and samples from women of child bearing age, showed levels over 30 ppb (Table III) and therefore these individuals had been in or approaching the fetal exposure risk range according to 1990 WHO guidelines which state "a 5% risk may be associated with a peak mercury level of 10-20 μg/g in maternal hair" (WHO, 1990:17). Using the 1:300 hair to blood conversion factor mentioned earlier this equates to 30-60 μg/L (ppb) in blood. A more detailed review of the cord blood results is shown in Figure 5. We can clearly see the downward trend of the cord blood levels over time. In Grassy Narrows, there were 156 cord blood samples taken in the 1978-92 period. The MeHg average level was 7.62 ppb (range = 1.5-72.7 sd = 9.89). In Whitedog, 153 samples were taken in the same period. The MeHg average level was 11.81 ppb (range = 1.5-125.2 sd = 17.76). The 1990 WHO MeHg criteria document also states "There is a need for epidemiological studies on children exposed in utero to levels of methylmercury that result in peak maternal hair mercury levels below 20 μg/g, in order to screen for those effects only detectable by available psychological and behavioural tests" (WHO, 1990:17). We therefore decided to try to assess the long term effects of fetal exposure in these communities, by looking at subtle developmental indicators.

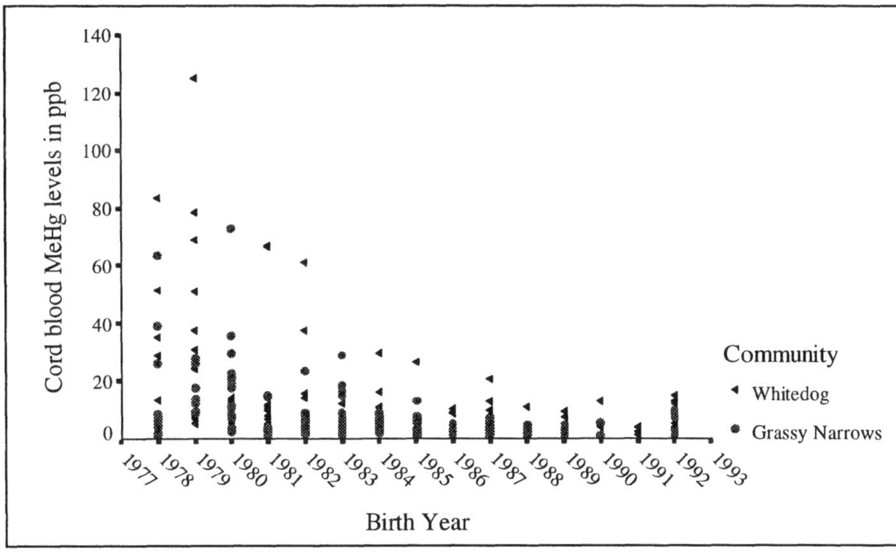

Fig. 5 Grassy Narrows and Whitedog MeHg in Cord Blood (1978-1992)

In the past, standard, but detailed, clinical examinations among Canadian First Nations people failed to prove abnormalities attributable to methylmercury (Wheatley *et al.*, 1979; Wheatley and Paradis, 1996) although one epidemiological study among the Cree of Quebec showed possible mild reflex abnormalities in Cree boys (McKeown-Eyssen and Ruedy, 1983). However these examinations did not look at possible neuropsychological and neurobehavioural effects. Many of the fetally exposed children in Grassy Narrows and Whitedog are now in secondary school. Therefore, stimulated by other international research projects on the effects of methylmercury on child development (Myers *et al.*, 1995; Weihe and Grandjean, 1996), we initiated a pilot project to attempt to assess the long term effects of methylmercury exposure on the neuropsychological development of those children whose fetal exposure we know from their cord blood methylmercury levels. The basic hypothesis, of course, was that higher methylmercury exposure of children leads to learning disabilities and impaired neuropsychological development. Although the potential for confounding factors was high due to the continuing social disruption in the communities, we felt that a window of opportunity existed to attempt this assessment. Falling community methylmercury levels and the children getting older and leaving school meant that the opportunity might not last very long. Early in 1995 we met with the community leaders to discuss a possible study. They were in agreement and therefore, with their support, we developed a program which includes four major components:

1. A school records review to assess general behaviour, attainment, attendance records and academic performance in various school disciplines..
2. Evaluation by teachers using the standardized Conners' (Conners' Rating Scale, 1969) and Achenbach's rating scales (Child Behavior Check List (CBCL),

Achenbach, 1991), specifically looking at behaviour including hyper-activity and aggressiveness.

3. An in-depth neuropsychological test battery focussing on factors such as memory, attention, executive functions, perceptual functions as well as basic sensory and motor functions.
4. A current hair sampling program to identify present methylmercury levels and compare to previous findings.

Grade	Grassy Narrows	Whitedog	Total
1	141 (54)	103 (27)	244 (81)
2	152 (62)	89 (27)	241 (89)
3	115 (45)	79 (22)	194 (67)
4	103 (44)	60 (21)	163 (65)
5	66 (30)	50 (19)	116 (49)
6	51 (21)	36 (11)	87 (32)
7	45 (19)	31 (7)	76 (26)
8	31 (10)	15 (8)	46 (18)
9	12 (5)	2 (1)	14 (6)

Table IV Available School Records: Total number of children for each grade (number with cord blood data)

In our assessment of the school records, we concentrated on subjects taught throughout the curriculum: mathematics, reading, writing and spelling. We also noted number of days late or absent. Table IV shows the total number of records for each grade and also the number of students for whom we had cord blood results.

Achenbach's Scale (CBCL)	Conner's Rating Scale
1. Working Hard	1. Hyperactivity
2. Appropriate Behaviour	2. Conduct Problem
3. Learning	3. Emotional-Indulgence
4. Happy	4. Anxious-Passive Problem
5. Four Adaptive Functioning Items	5. Asocial
6. Withdrawn Scale	6. Daydream-Attention Problem
7. Somatic Complaints Scale	7. Hyperactivity Index
8. Anxious/Depressed Scale	
9. Social Problems Scale	
10. Thought Problems Scale	
11. Attention Problems Scale	
12. Aggressive Behaviour Scale	
13. Internalizing	
14. Externalizing	
15. Score for Total Problems	

Fig. 6 Achenbach's and Conner's Rating Scale components

The CBCL (Figure 6) is a standardized, effective test of behaviour used extensively in schools in North America and covers an assessment of a wide range of behaviour patterns. The Conners Test (Figure 6) has a specific emphasis on hyperactivity. It overlaps to some extent with the CBCL but the two tests are frequently carried out together to complement and confirm findings. Both tests were carried out in Grassy Narrows and Whitedog by teachers who best knew the children.

The neuropsychological sensory / motor test battery (Figure 7) is comprised of a wide range of tests which were carried out by four trained psychologists working at the schools on the two reserves.

1. Basic Motor Tests
2. Global Motor Tests
3. Basic Sensory Examination
   - a) Vision
   - b) Audition
   - c) Somatosensory Tests
     - c.1 Stereognosis
     - c.2 Somatognosy
     - c.3 Face-Hand Test
     - c.4 Finger Agnosia
     - c.5 Two-point discrimination test
   - d) Olfaction: Smell Identification test
4. Mood / Affect
5. Memory
   - a) Immediate Verbal Recall
   - b) Episodic Memory
   - c) Delayed Verbal Recall
   - d) Immediate Visuo-Spatial Memory
   - e) Delayed Visuo-Spatial Memory
6. Attention
   - a) WISC-III Freedom From Distractibility Factor
   - b) WISC-III Speed of Perceptual Processing
   - c) The Conners and Achenbach Subscores on Attention
7. Social Behaviour
8. Learning
9. Visuo-Spatial Tasks
   - a) The Reproduction of the Rey Complex Figure
   - b) Block Design & Object Assembly from the WISC-III
10. Visual Perception
    - a) Picture Completion of the WISC-III
    - b) Gestalt-Closure test
11. Motor Skills
    - a) Purdue Pegboard
    - b) Subtest from the McCarthy Scale of children's abilities
12. Communication Skills
    - a) Verbal Communication from the WISC-III
    - b) Phonetics & Semantic Verbal Fluency Tests
    - c) Riddles from the Kaufman ABC
13. Quantitative Abilities
    - a) Math Results
    - b) Arithmetic of the WISC-III
14. Executive Control, Activity Regulation, Problem Solving
    - a) Kaufman Hand Movement Test
    - b) Mazes from the WISC-III
    - c) Picture Arrangement from the WISC-III
    - d) Luria's Seriations

Fig. 7 Neuropsychological Sensory/Motor test battery

Hair samples were taken from the children to ascertain current mercury levels. Most children now have very low levels and all are below 20 ppb. There was good cooperation by the communities as shown by the number of parental consents (177 from Whitedog and 145 from Grassy Narrows). Teachers completed 243 CBCL and 250 Conners assessments and 181 neuropsychological testing batteries were carried out by the four psychologists by June of 1996. Two hundred seventy six school records are being reviewed. The data analysis is presently underway. With community agreement, we propose to enlarge our parameters to include pregnancy and mother and child medical histories.

3. Conclusion

In an international context, residents of the Canadian aboriginal communities of Grassy Narrows and Whitedog have been, in the recent past, among the groups most highly exposed to elevated levels of methylmercury in fish. With changes in the process at the pulp and paper mill, mercury has not been released into the English-Wabigoon river system for a number of years and mercury levels in fish are falling (Government of Ontario, 1993). Of more immediate importance to us is that the levels in the residents of the two communities have also been falling. Analysis of the twenty year data base as well as recent testing have confirmed this fact. However, there remain many problems in the communities due to the social disruption produced by the changes in lifestyle resulting from the inability to subsistence fish and the lack of opportunity to guide sport fishermen. However, with the on-going concern regarding fetal exposure to methylmercury we felt that this possibility to utilize known cord blood methylmercury levels of children currently at school on the reserves represented a window of opportunity which we should take. The numbers of children available for the study are not quite as high as we had initially anticipated and the cord blood levels in the available group are somewhat lower than we had expected. Also, there are a large number of potential confounders. However, a great deal of neuropsychological and behavioural data has now been collected and we intend to try to supplement that, as indicated. It is our hope that when analysis is complete the information will at least add to the total knowledge base on subtle developmental indicators of fetal methylmercury exposure and may make a useful contribution to this difficult area, especially when taken into consideration with the other fetal methylmercury exposure studies under way elsewhere in the world. Our target is to report our findings within the next year.

Acknowledgements

The authors wish to gratefully acknowledge the First Nations people of Grassy Narrows and Whitedog with whose cooperation and on whose behalf this work has been and is being carried out. Funding (in part) is from the Health Canada Action Plan on Health and the Environment (Green Plan).

References

Achenbach, T.M. (1991). *Manual for the Teacher's Report Form and 1991 Profile.* Burlington, VT: University of Vermont Department of Psychiatry.

Bishop, J.N., and Neary, B.P.: 1976, *Mercury levels in Fish from Northwestern Ontario 1970-1975.* Ontario Ministry of the Environment, Toronto.

Conners, C.K.: 1969, A teacher rating scale for use in doing studies with children. *AM. J. of Psychiatry* 126, 884-888.

Erikson, K.: 1994, *A New Species of Trouble: Explorations of Disaster, Trauma, and Community.* W.W. Norton and Co, New York.

Farant, J.P., Brissette, D., Moncion, L., Bigras, L., and Chartrand, A.: 1981, Improved cold-vapor atomic absorption technique for the microdetermination of total and inorganic mercury in biological samples. *J. Anal. Toxicol.* 5,47-51.

Government of Ontario, 1993. Guide to eating Ontario Sport Fish.

McKeown-Eyssen, E.E., and Ruedy, J.:1983, Prevalence of neurological abnormality in Cree Indians exposed to methylmercury in northern Quebec. *Clin. Inves. Med.* 6,161-169.

Myers, G. J., Davidson, W., Cox, C., Shamlaye, C. F., Tanner, M. A., Marsh, D. O., Cernichiari, E., Lapham, L. W., Berlin, M., Clarkson, T. W.: 1995, Summary of the

Seychelles Child Development Study on the Relationship of Fetal Methylmercury Exposure to Neurodevelopment. *NeuroToxicology* 16(4), 711-715.

Phelps, R. W., Clarkson, T.W., Kershaw, T.G., and Wheatley, B.: 1980, Interrelationships of blood and hair mercury concentrations in a North American population exposed to methylmercury. *Arch. Environ. Health* 35,161-168.

Rudd, J. W. M., Turner, M. A., Furutani, A., Swick, A. L., and Townsend, B.E.: 1983, The English-Wabigoon River system: I. A synthesis of recent research with a view towards mercury amelioration. *Can. J. Fish. Aquat. Sci.* 40, 2206-2217.

Shkilnyk, A.M.: 1985, *A Poison Stronger than Love: The Destruction of an Ojibwa Community*, New Haven, Yale University Press.

Weihe, P., Grandjean, P., Debes, F., White, R.: 1996, Health implications for Faroe Islanders of heavy metals and PCBs from pilot whales. *Science of the Total Environment* 186, 141-148

Wheatley, B.: 1979, *Methylmercury in Canada: Exposure of Indian and Inuit residents to Methylmercury in the Canadian Environment.* Department of National Health and Welfare, Medical Services Branch, Ottawa. 200pp

Wheatley, B., Barbeau, A., Clarkson, T. W., and Lapham, L.: 1979, Methylmercury poisoning in Canadian Indians - The elusive diagnosis. *Can. J. Neurol. Sci.* 6(4), 417-422.

Wheatley, B., Paradis, S.: 1996, Balancing human exposure, risk and reality: Questions raised by the Canadian Aboriginal methylmercury program. *NeuroToxicology.* 17(1), 241-250.

Wheatley, B., Paradis, S.: 1995, Exposure of Canadian Aboriginal peoples to methymercury. *Water, Air and Soil Pollution.* 80, 3-11.

Wheatley, M. A.: 1996, The importance of social and cultural effects of mercury on Aboriginal peoples. *NeuroToxicology.* 17(1), 251-256

WHO: 1990, *Environmental Health Criteria 101. Methylmercury.* World Health Organisation, Geneva.

WHO: 1976, *Environmental Health Criteria I. Mercury.* World Health Organisation, Geneva.

MERCURY IN NORTHERN QUÉBEC: ROLE OF THE MERCURY AGREEMENT AND STATUS OF RESEARCH AND MONITORING

GASTON CHEVALIER [1,2], CHARLES DUMONT [1,3]
CLAUDE LANGLOIS [1,4], AND ALAN PENN [1,5]

[1] *James Bay Mercury Committee, Montréal,*
[2] *Université du Québec à Montréal,* C.P. 8888, Succ. "Centre-Ville", *Montréal,* Québec, H3C 3P8
[3] *Cree Board of Health and Social Services of James Bay,* 1610, Ste-Catherine ouest, Montréal, Québec, H3H 2S2
[4] *Vice-présidence Environnement, Hydro-Québec,* 75 René-Lévesque ouest, *Montréal,* Québec, H2Z 1A4
[5] *Cree Regional Authority,* 277 Duke street, *Montréal,* Québec, H3C 2M2

ABSTRACT. In order to determine the nature and extent of the problem caused by the presence of mercury in the environment of the James Bay territory a Mercury Agreement was signed in 1986 jointly by the Crees, the Government of Québec and Hydro-Québec. The objectives were to minimize potential hazards to human health arising from the presence of mercury in the environment, to alleviate negative impacts on the Crees, their way of life and their harvesting activities and to provide for remedial measures. Monitoring of mercury concentrations in fish show that, 15 years after impounding of La Grande-2 reservoir, the concentrations remain higher in reservoirs than in natural lakes but they are now decreasing in both predatory (Northern pike) and non-predatory (Whitefish) fishes. Monitoring of the mercury exposure among the Crees showed that concentrations in hair have decreased and are now stabilized, for most of the population, to concentrations that do not present a health risk. This decrease may be attributed to a reduction in fish consumption and/or a possible switch of the diet towards non-piscivorous fish, less contaminated by mercury.

1. Introduction

Environmental and health concerns about mercury appeared among Northern Québec Cree communities in the early 1970's, following contamination of fish due to effluents from a kraft mill containing a chlor-alkali plant (Berkes *et al.* ; 1972). Subsequent surveys revealed elevated exposure to methylmercury in Cree communities throughout Northwestern Québec (Santé et Bien-Être Social Canada, 1979). This exposure was attributed mainly to the consumption of fish from inland waters, often remote from localized sources. Approximately onc half of thc adult population over the age of 35 underwent neurological assessments, as well as a cohort of 300 children exposed in utero (Mckeown-Eyssen and Ruedy, 1983a, 1983b, Mckeown-Eyssen, Ruedy and Neims 1983). Measures were taken to limit the subsistence fishery and subsequent fish consumption has remained well below levels recorded in the early 1970's (Weinstein and Penn, 1987).

These concerns were revived in some communities affected by the hydroelectric development of the La Grande Complex, which has created large reservoirs by empoundment of approximately 11 500 square kilometers of land. In order to determine the nature and extent of the problem caused by the presence of mercury in the environment of the James Bay territory, with particular reference to the La Grande Hydroelectric Complex (Figure 1), a Mercury Agreement was signed in 1986 jointly by the Crees, the Government of Québec and Hydro-Québec (C.Q. H.-Q., 1986). The implementation of this Agreement is under the responsibility of

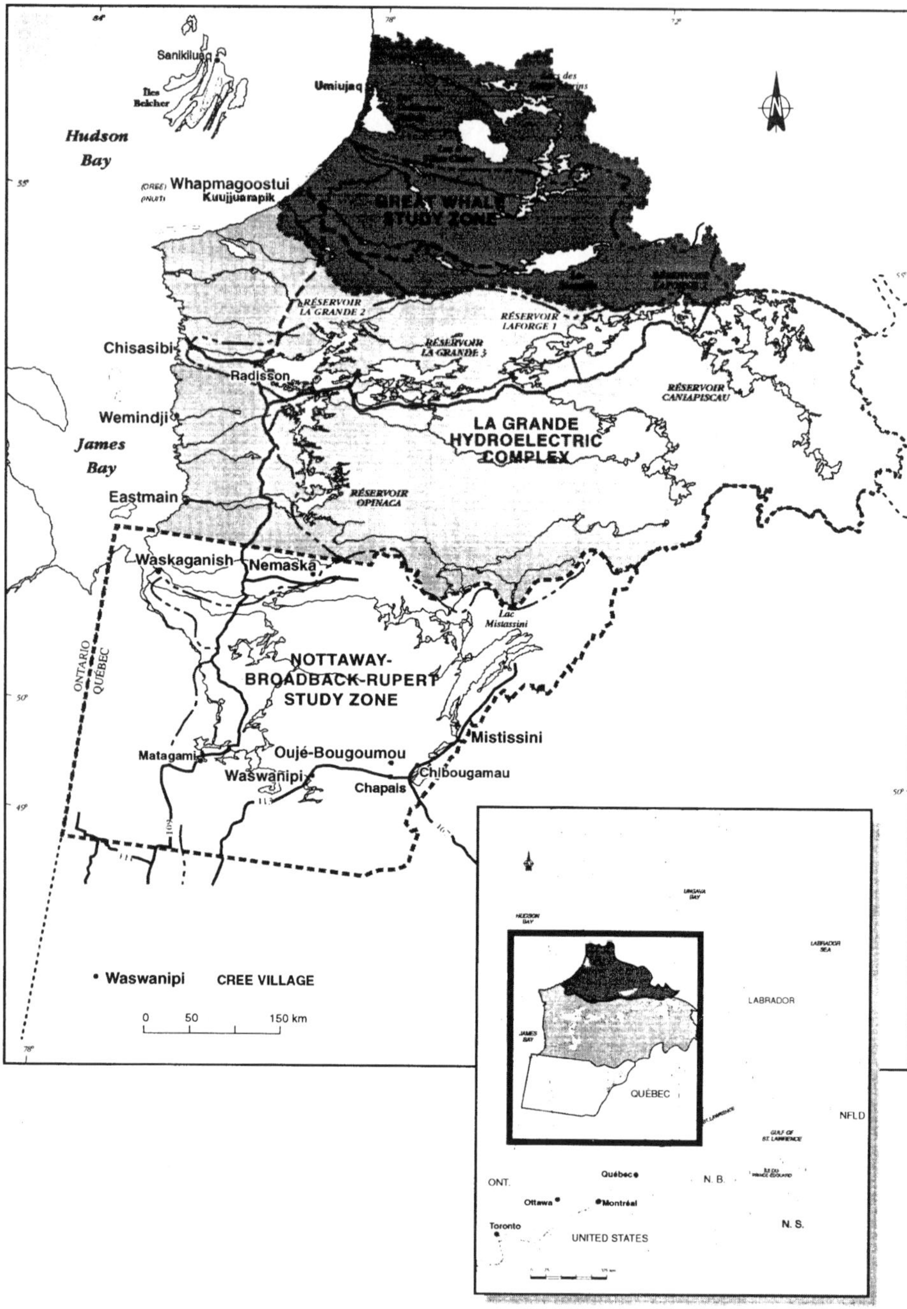

Fig. 1. Location of Study Areas in Northern Québec

the James Bay Mercury Committee, made up of representatives of the above-mentioned authorities and whose chairman was appointed by the Québec Government .

The objectives of this Agreement were to minimize potential hazards to human health arising from the presence of mercury in the environment, to alleviate any existing and potential negative impacts on the Crees, their way of life and their harvesting activities and to provide for remedial measures to reduce the release of mercury into the environment. The Mercury Agreement program includes monitoring of mercury in fish, monitoring of the Crees exposure to mercury, study of social and economic impacts of mercury on the Crees and implementation of remedial measures to enable the Crees to continue to carry out their harvesting activities and way of life. In order to improve our knowledge and understanding of the phenomenon of increased mercury in hydroelectric reservoirs and of the long term potential risk for public health, the Agreement also includes research activities on environment and health issues related to mercury (James Bay Mercury Committee, 1995a).

2. Mercury in fish and wildlife

The monitoring of mercury concentrations in fish has been conducted by Hydro-Québec in the La Grande Complex since 1978. The species considered included those most consumed by the Cree inhabitants of the territory, such as Lake Whitefish (*Coregonus clupeaformis*), Cisco (*Coregonus artedii*), Lake Trout (*Salvelinus namaycush*), Northern Pike (*Esox lucius*), Walleye (*Stizostedion vitreum*) and Longnose Sucker (*Catostomus catostomus*).

Hydro-Québec observed in 1982 increasing levels of mercury in fish from the oldest reservoir, the La Grande 2 reservoir, where the maximum levels reached from 3.5 to 5 times the pre-impoundment levels in the various species of fish (Brouard *et al.* ; 1990). The results obtained in 1994 show that, 15 years after impounding of the La Grande-2 reservoir, the mercury concentrations in fish remain higher in reservoirs than in natural lakes for most species (Schetagne *et al.* ; 1996) However, the mercury levels are now decreasing or stabilized in both non-predatory (Whitefish) and predatory (Northern pike) fish (Figures 2 and 3).

In natural areas of Northern Québec unaffected by hydroelectric development, numerous piscivorous species of fish and wildlife also show significant concentrations of mercury in flesh (Table I). In some tissues, the concentrations measured were much higher than those observed in muscle, particulary in feathers and livers of Common mergansers (*Mergus Merganser*) and Herring gulls (*Larus argentatus*) (Langlois et al, 1995).

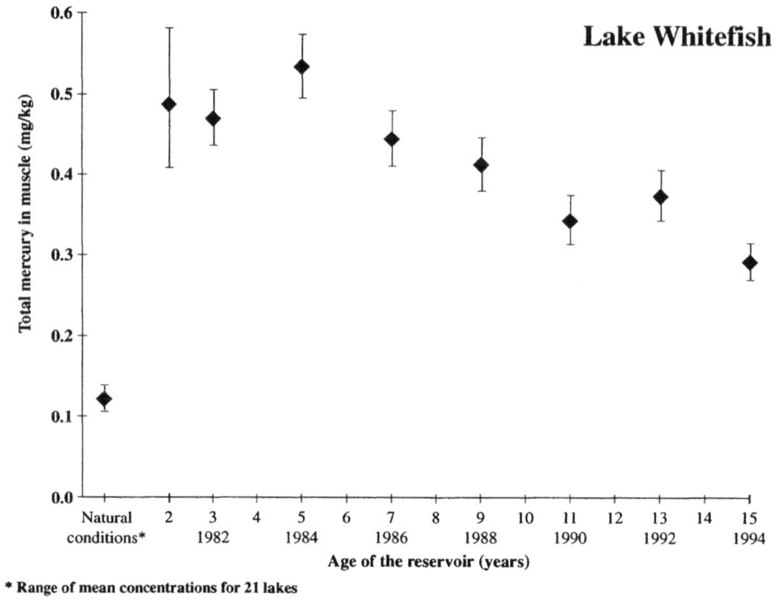

Fig. 2. Mercury Concentrations in Lake Whitefish from the La Grande-2 Reservoir (Standardized Length of 400 mm) and 95 % Mean Confidence Interval

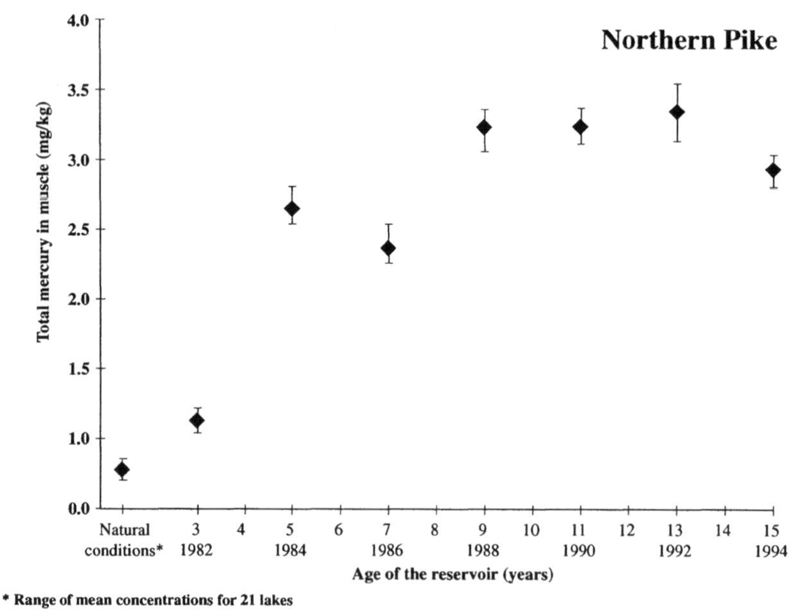

Fig. 3. Mercury Concentrations in Northern Pike from the La Grande 2 Reservoir (Standardized Length of 700 mm) and 95 % Mean Confidence Interval

Table I

Levels of Total Mercury (mg/kg Fresh Weight) in Various Tissues of Selected Wildlife Species

	Great Whale				Nottaway-Broadback-Rupert			
Species	Mean	±	S.D.	N	Mean	±	S.D.	N
Northern pike (muscle)	0,63	±	0,46	75	0,93	±	0,51	636
Walleye (muscle)	-		-	-	0,78	±	0,46	789
Lake trout (muscle)	0,77	±	0,66	504	-		-	-
Common merganser								
• muscle	1,27	±	0,48	13	1,41	±	1,26	19
• liver	17,53	±	12,06	13	10,9	±	7,5	15
• feathers	9,97	±	2,88	12	7,31	±	2,91	15
Herring gull								
• muscle	1,03	±	0,80	28	1,59	±	1,32	13
• liver	2,91	±	2,35	27	3,63	±	2,52	13
• feathers	11,54	±	8,55	27	19,1	±	15,3	13
American mink								
• muscle	2,40	±	2,24	6			-	-

Adapted from Langlois et *al*, 1995

3. Mercury exposure among the Crees

The Cree exposure to mercury was monitored by Health and Welfare Canada from 1971 to 1978. Since 1982, the Cree Board of Health and Social Services of James Bay (CBHSSJB) is concentrating the surveillance among specific groups of the population, namely the women of childbearing age, the pregnant women and their newborns and the people over 40 years of age who tend to have a more traditional way of life and who consume the most fish (Dumont *et al.* ; 1988).

In recent years, mercury concentrations in hair have decreased and are now stabilized, for most of the population, to concentrations that do not present a health risk (Dumont *et al.* ; 1996). The results obtained in 1993 and 1994 from inland and coastal communities, where a total of 3 599 individuals were sampled, reveal that 90% of the children between 4 and 19 years old have mercury concentrations in hair lower than 2.5 mg/kg and 90% of the persons of all age groups have concentrations lower than 22 mg/kg (Figure 4). Among the men and women aged 40 and over, the number of persons showing high concentrations has decreased significantly in the last ten years, revealing in 1994 only 12 persons exceeding the intervention threshold of 30 mg/kg established by the Cree Board of Health and Social Services of James Bay (Figure 5). Similarly, in 1993 and 1994, all the women of childbearing age (15-39 years old) showed concentrations of mercury lower than the intervention threshold of 15 mg/kg (upper limit of acceptable level) used by the CBHSSJB.

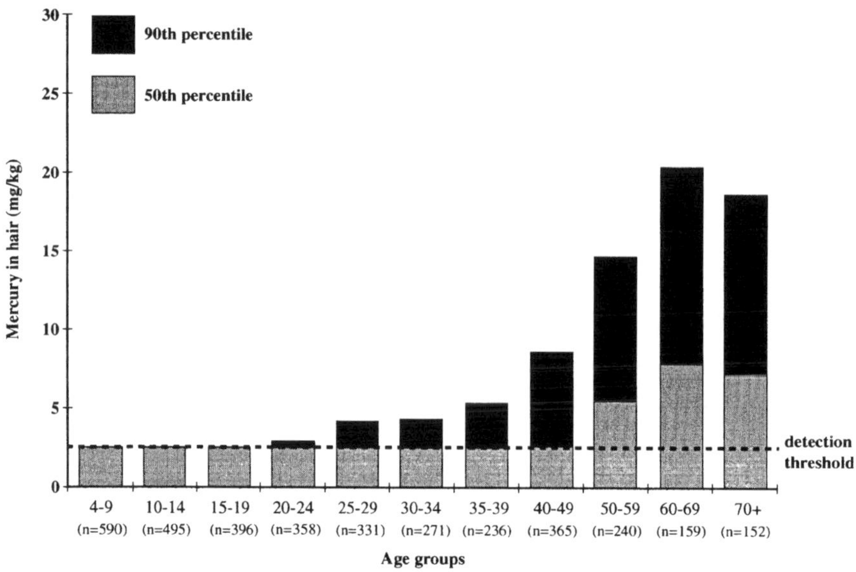

Fig. 4. Mercury Concentrations in Hair (90th and 50th Percentile) According to Age Groups for the 9 Cree Communities in 1993 - 1994

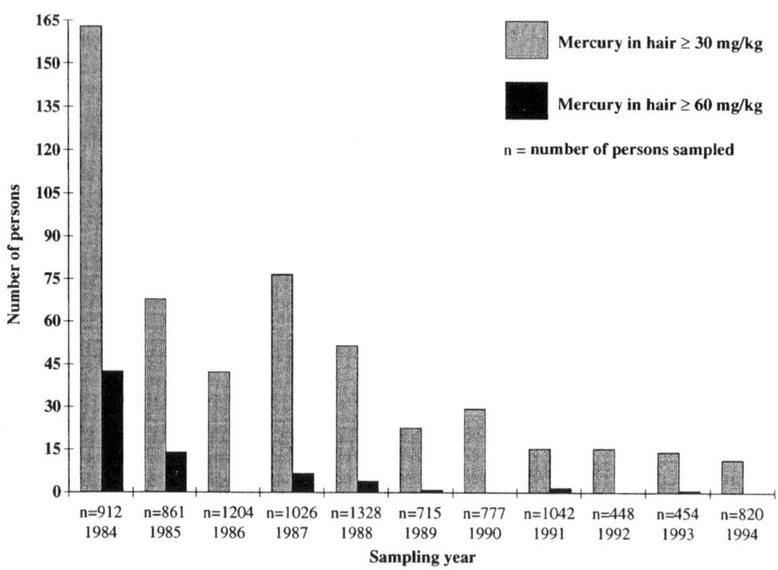

Fig. 5. Number of Persons (Men and Women 40 Years and Over) from the 9 Cree Communities Showing High Levels of Mercury Exposure

The results also indicate that 90% of the mothers showed mercury concentrations in hair, at time of childbirth, lower than 4 mg/kg in 1991, as compared with a 90th percentile of 12 mg/kg in 1983 (Figure 6) (Girard and Dumont, 1995). The concentrations in umbilical cord blood showed similar trends, decreasing from a 90th percentile of 90 ug/L in 1983 to a 90th percentile of 12 ug/L in 1991 (Figure 7). The decrease is also confirmed among trappers and non-trappers groups when we examine the mercury concentrations of persons sampled both in 1988 and in 1993/94 (Table II).

Table II

Comparison of Mercury Concentrations in the Hair of People Sampled Both in 1988 and 1993 - 1994

Population group	N	Year	50th percentile	90th percentile	Maximum
TRAPPERS					
Women (15-39 years)	96	1988	2,5 [2]	5,8	25,3
	96	1993-94 [1]	2,5	4,6	10,1
Men and Women	361	1988	8,4	22,1	85,6
(40 years and over)	361	1993-94	7,3	17,8	42,2
ALL	457	1988	7,0	20,8	85,6
	457	1993-94	5,1	16,4	42,2
NON TRAPPERS					
Women (15-39 years)	318	1988	2,5	4,4	13,9
	318	1993-94	2,5	3,3	12,4
Men + Women	303	1988	5,8	17,4	41,3
(40 years and over)	303	1993-94	3,5	11,2	24,1
ALL	621	1988	2,9	12,8	41,3
	621	1993-94	2,5	8,1	24,1

1 Sampled in 1993 in inland communities and in 1994 in coastal communities.
2 The detection limit of the laboratory is 2.5 mg/kg.

This decrease is attributed to a reduction in fish consumption and/or a possible switch of the diet towards non-piscivorous fish, less contaminated by mercury. It is also possible that this very limited fish consumption is only temporary among the young people who, as adults, may become more regular consumers of fish. In view of the nutritional value of fish, its health benefits for the Crees and its sizable economic and sociocultural importance, the Cree Board of Health and Social Services of James Bay recommends that aboriginal populations eat fish at least twice a week, with particular emphasis on non predatory species (James Bay Mercury Committee, 1995b). As part of the Mercury Agreement, several information campaigns were conducted in the Cree communities. In order to maximize the success of such campaigns, the information tools , including posters, brochures, radio programs, public meetings or videos, were presented in the Cree language.

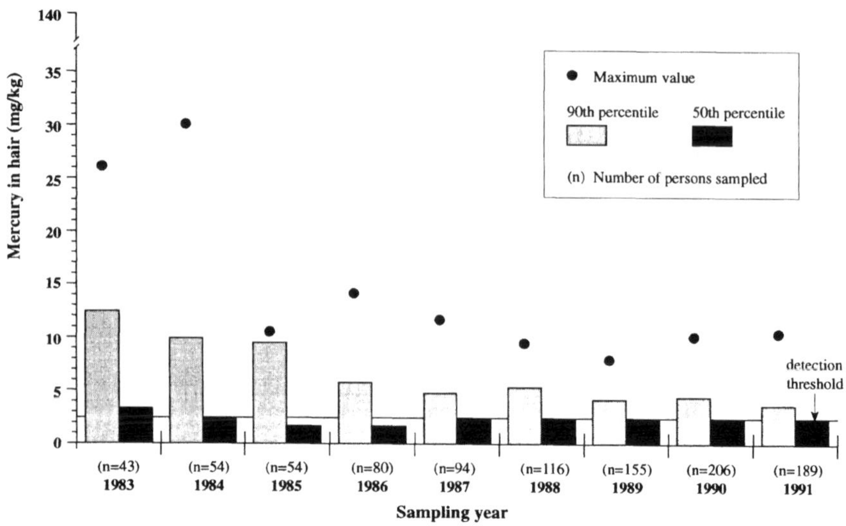

Fig. 6. Mercury Concentrations in Mothers' Hair at Time of Delivery: Percentile and Maximum Values

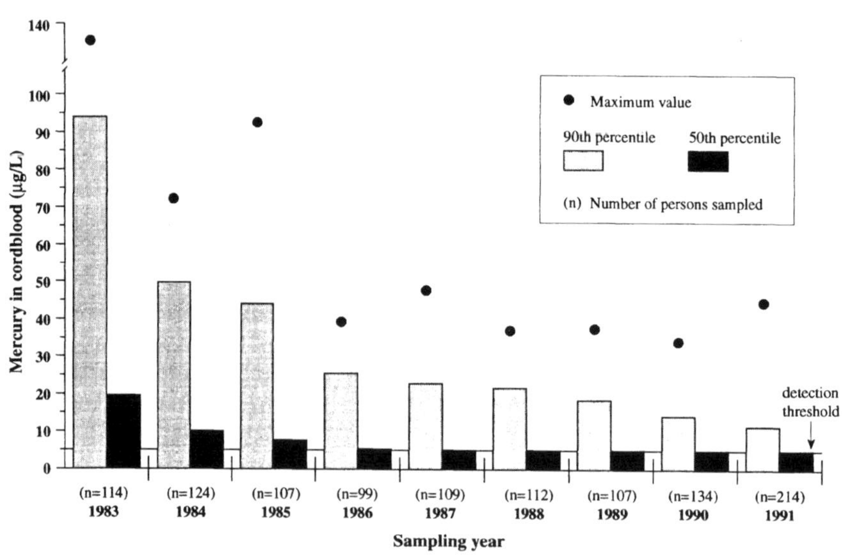

Note : approximate number of live births per year : 257 to 300.

Fig. 7. Mercury Concentrations in Newborns' Cord Blood: Percentile and Maximum Values

4. Remedial Measures

Remedial measures were undertaken with the Cree communities directly affected by the hydro-electric development to allow them to continue their harvesting activities as much as possible. These measures include supporting fisheries in areas where fish is less contaminated, such as in coastal waters where some communities have developed communal coastal fisheries. Since 1989, the community of Wemindji has harvested more than 70 000 fishes from three coastal camps, of which 72 % were Lake whitefish, 21 % were Cisco and 7 % were Speckled trout (Tremblay and Langlois, 1996). These fishes were distributed from house to house in the community, which ensured free access to valuable fish meal for all groups of the community. Appropriate biological monitoring of the fisheries is encouraged by the Committee in order to avoid overharvesting of the fishing sites. For this purpose, the Cree Regional Authority and Hydro-Québec provide scientific and technical help to the Cree communities.

Mercury Agreement funding was also used to support a demonstration project for the artificial reproduction of sturgeon (Branchaud et al, 1996). This species is particularly vulnerable to overharvesting and the La Grande complex is located at its northern limit of distribution. In the longer term, techniques of artificial reproduction and protection of young-of-the-year could be used to augment natural recruitment, and possibly re-introduce the species in areas where its survival may be compromised.

In other communities, some projects supported enhancement of wildlife habitats in alternate sites or for alternative species. In the community of Chisasibi, the tallymen of several traplines thus created new goose pounds or improved existing sites by appropriate forest and brush clearing, in order to make these environments more attractive to waterfowl and improve hunting success.

5. Conclusion

Mercury monitoring in the environment of the la Grande complex should continue until the levels measured in fish from the reservoirs are comparable to those measured in fish from the adjacent natural lakes. Policies for screening the Cree population are being reassessed in the light of the 1993 and 1994 surveys and of the generalized decline observed in mercury exposure. An investigation following the harvesting of fish from inland lakes showed rapid increases in exposure to mercury of people from the coastal community of Eastmain (Girard *et al.* ; 1996). Further surveillance of the Cree population, or of selected groups, may be necessary if there is a renewal of inland fishing.

The remedial measures implemented with the communities have contributed to reduce mercury exposure among the Crees, while encouraging the carrying out of traditional fishing and hunting activities. These measures represent an attempt to contribute to the acquisition by the Cree communities of suitable expertise and basic equipment to allow resources harvesting and proper management in a context of sustainable development. The future of subsistence fishing is a continuing source of concern and further work will be needed to ensure its survival. This is especially important in the light of the growing evidence for the protection rôle of fish in human disease.

6. Acknowledgments

We wish to thank the Cree people for their cooperation with the various activities undertaken in the context of the Mercury Agreement. We also thank all participants from Hydro-Québec, the Cree Regional Authority and the Cree Board of Health and Social Services of James Bay who participated in the various studies or activities.

References

Berkes et al, 1972. Environmental aspects of the pulp and paper industry in Québec. Montréal : Terra Nova

Branchaud, A., A.D. Gendron, C. Lemire et R. Dion (1996). Reproduction artificielle de l'esturgeon jaune dans le nord du Québec. Rapport présenté par l'Université du Québec à Montréal, GVL Environnement et l'Administration régionale crie au Comité de la Baie James sur le mercure, Montréal, 24 pp.

Brouard, D., C. Demers, R. Lalumière, R. Schetagne et R. Verdon (1990). Rapport synthèse. Évolution des teneurs en mercure des poissons du complexe hydroélectrique La Grande, Québec (1978-1990). Rapport conjoint vice-présidence Environnement, Hydro-Québec et Groupe Environnement Shooner inc. 100 pp.

C.Q.H.-Q. (1986). Mercury Agreement. Text of the Agreement. Montréal, Québec. 16 sections and one appendix.

Dumont, C. , F. Noël and M. Girard (1996). Change in the mercury exposure of the Crees of James Bay (Québec), submitted for publication.

Dumont, C., R. Wilkins, T. Kosatsky and S. Lapierre (1988). Arctic Medical Research, No 47, suppl. 1: 168-174.

Girard, M. and C. Dumont (1995). Water, Air and Soil Pollution, 80:13-19.

Girard, M., F. Noël and C. Dumont (1996). Arctic Medical Research; 55:69-74.

James Bay Mercury Committee (1995a). Report of Activities, 1993-1994. James Bay Mercury Committee, Montréal, 48 pp.

James Bay Mercury Committee (1995b). Mercury, Questions and Answers. Brochure and posters prepared by the Cree Board of Health and Social Services of James Bay, Hydro-Québec and the Cree Regional Authority for the James Bay Mercury Committee. Montréal, 24 pp and 13 posters.

Langlois, C., R. Langis et M. Pérusse, (1995). Water, Air and Soil Pollution, 80 : 1021-1024

Mckeown-Eyssen, G.E. and Ruedy, J. (1983a). American Journal of Epidemiology, 118(4):461-469.

Mckeown-Eyssen, G.E. and Ruedy, J. (1983b). Clinical and Investigative Medicine, 6(3): 161-169.

Mckeown-Eyssen, G.E.,J. Ruedy and A. Neims (1983). American Journal of Epidemiology, 118(4):470-479.

Santé et Bien-Être Social Canada (1979). Le méthylmercure au Canada. Exposition des Indiens et des Inuits au méthylmercure présent dans l'environnement canadien. Ministère de la Santé et du Bien-Être Social du Canada, Direction des Services Médicaux, Ottawa.

Schetagne, R., R. Verdon, C. Langlois and J.F. Doyon (1996). Mercury evolution (1978-1995) in fishes of the La Grande Hydroelectric Complex, Québec, Canada. Communication presented at the 4th International Conference on Mercury as a Global Pollutant, Hamburg, Germany, August 4-8 1996, 12 pp.

Tremblay, A. et C. Langlois (1996). Mesures d'atténuation réalisées avec les communautés cries de la Baie James de 1989 à 1995 dans le cadre de la Convention sur le Mercure. Rapport présenté au Comité de la Baie James sur le Mercure par la vice-présidence Environnement d'Hydro-Québec, Montréal, 44 pp.

Weinstein, M. and A. Penn (1987). Mercury and the Chisasibi fishery: A report prepared for the Cree Regional Authority. Cree Regional Authority, Montréal.

SOCIAL AND CULTURAL IMPACTS OF MERCURY POLLUTION ON ABORIGINAL PEOPLES IN CANADA

MARGARET A. WHEATLEY

Eco-Anth Consulting, 32 Windfield Crescent, Kanata, Ontario, K2M 2B7, Canada

Abstract Among Aboriginal peoples in Canada, mercury pollution has had an impact on social and cultural well being, both at the community level and among individual members within the community, even when there are no provable direct health effects. This paper explores the link between mercury pollution and social and cultural disruption in Canadian Aboriginal communities. It demonstrates how factors such as Aboriginal holistic concepts of environment and health, perceptions, and difficulties in communication can contribute to indirect impacts of mercury pollution on health and well being. It is argued that, given the blood mercury levels among Canadian Aboriginal peoples, social and cultural impacts of mercury pollution present a much greater problem than do the direct clinical effects of exposure.

1. Introduction

Environmental mercury pollution, often the result of Western industrial development, has had a major impact on Canadian Aboriginal people, who frequently receive few of the benefits of such activity, while suffering the most disruption to their lifestyles. Even when there are no provable direct health effects from exposure to mercury, Aboriginal peoples' holistic concept of health leads them to regard social and cultural disruption which results from the pollution as being a direct effect on health. In addition, the concept of balance and harmony, and the inter-relatedness of health and environment in Aboriginal peoples' world views exacerbates these effects (Wheatley, M.A, 1994) Various factors play a role in this process, but this paper focusses on how: a) Aboriginal concepts of environment and health; b) perceptions; and c) difficulties in communication contribute to social and cultural impacts and their subsequent health effects. Three Canadian Aboriginal communities are used as examples.

2. Aboriginal Holistic Concepts of Environment and Health

Aboriginal concepts of the environment encompass its inter-connected elements. Aboriginal people perceive themselves to be an integral part of the environment (Berger, 1977), "part of the land, part of the water" (Yukon Elder, cited in McClellan, 1987:333). People's place in the environment and the philosophy of environmental harmony is expressed in the words of Chief Seattle's statement of 1854: "The earth does not belong to man; man belongs to the earth....Man did not weave the web of life; he is merely a strand in it. Whatever he does to the web, he does to himself". For Aboriginal peoples depending on environmental resources for survival, respectful behaviour towards the environment is perceived as being necessary to ensure the maintenance of good health.

Aboriginal understandings of health are therefore inseparable from their concept of environment (Wheatley, M.A., 1994; 1995), with health representing balance among all the inter-connected aspects of well being. This balance is perceived in the close relationship

Aboriginal peoples have to the environment in which they live. Cultural identity is expressed in traditional values, such as respect, caring, sharing and responsibility for oneself and others. The harvesting and consumption of natural resources enhances peoples' feelings of well being, acting as a tonic and allowing communication with nature. People dependent on the environment for their survival were, and are, in turn responsible for maintaining a healthy environment, so that it can support the future generations for whom they feel responsible (Wheatley, 1996). A closely related factor is that of perceptions.

3. Perceptions

Perceptions are very real for the people concerned. Risks appear greater when they are perceived to be unfairly shared, are imposed on individuals or not easily controlled, or are linked to man-made hazards (Slovic *et al.*, 1982). Aboriginal people's view that the environment which they respect has been violated heightens this effect. Difficulties in understanding the concept of "invisible" contaminants and their effects influence perceptions, which are based on holistic concepts of health and environment. They determine what people believe to be the danger and the actions taken to reduce the perceived risk (Wheatley, M.A., 1995). Perceptions may differ from the measured risk and are little influenced by scientific assessments and statements which are difficult to believe or understand. As a result, mercury in the environment may be linked to changes in physical health, even when there is no proven link. Perceptions of risk may over-ride the actual risk, resulting in reactions which may produce real health consequences (Wheatley, 1996). Perceptions may also be influenced by difficulties in communication.

4. Communication

Aboriginal traditional knowledge is based on an individual's cumulative experience, incorporating traditional concepts of environment and health. This may lead to difficulties when communicating with people with different backgrounds. When subsistence resources are affected by contaminants such as mercury, the people depending on these resources need to know. However, the language and method of communication must be simple and clear, explaining why tests are needed and what they can and cannot do to provide answers (Wheatley, M.A., 1995). When results or advice are provided, scientific language such as "tolerable daily intake" should be replaced by non-technical language, such as "number of fish meals per week". Good communication may help to moderate the social and cultural effects if it helps to reassure communities if there is no risk, prevent panic if there is a possible risk, or justify advisory notices if they are necessary. Mis-communication or poor communication, by scientists or media, can have real health consequences if it reinforces erroneous perceptions (Wheatley, 1996).

Responses seen in three Canadian Aboriginal communities exposed to environmental methylmercury provide examples to illustrate these points.

GRASSY NARROWS AND WHITEDOG

During the 1960s, residents of the Indian reserves of Grassy Narrows and Whitedog on the English-Wabigoon river system in Northwestern Ontario were exposed to mercury from an upstream chlor-alkali plant. By 1970, high levels of mercury in fish led to the closure of the commercial fishery which, with guiding, provided an economic base, in addition to subsistence fishing. Fishing was part of their cultural identity, an integrative social activity in which everyone had a role and where traditional skills were passed on. Difficulty in understanding high mercury levels in both fish and humans created anxiety among the residents of the two reserves. Media attention and conflicting information from different sources increased their perception of the risk (Erikson, 1994). Some of the highest human mercury levels in Canada were found there (Wheatley and Paradis, 1995). In addition to the potential health risk, the environment was perceived to be poisoned and this increased their concern. People could no longer rely on their traditional knowledge and skills to guide them. Social disruption ensued (Shkilnyk, 1985; Erikson, 1994). In both communities police reported widespread family violence, child neglect, solvent sniffing by children as young as six and an increase in violent deaths during the early 1970s. Grassy Narrows (population 400) recorded 31 violent deaths, including 5 suicides, in the years 1974-1978, most alcohol related (Erikson, 1994). Even after compensation was paid social problems persisted, especially in Whitedog, where solvents are smuggled into the community and 4 suicides were reported in the spring of 1995 (Guttormson, 1995). Both communities reflected the hopelessness which results from the destruction of a familiar lifestyle, loss of self-esteem because of an inability to provide, and loss of traditional values of respect, sharing and caring. What was originally a potential health problem because of the high mercury levels in the local fish became a much greater social and cultural problem. Aboriginal concepts of health and environment no longer provided answers where there was a very real risk. Their perceptions of the risk were increased by conflicting or confusing information from media, scientists and health care personnel.

SALLUIT

Salluit, an Inuit community, lies on the Hudson Strait in Northern Quebec. In the late 1970s, several residents were found to have high mercury levels. Before the people in the community had been properly informed, a media report erroneously referred to Minamata disease, which requires human mercury levels an order of magnitude higher than had been found in Salluit (Wheatley, B. 1995). As a result of the fear and concern that this report caused, the whole community stopped eating the country food on which it depended. The extent of this dependence was reflected in harvesting data (James Bay and Northern Quebec Native Harvesting Research Committee, 1979). Affordable alternative foods were limited (Wheatley and Wheatley, 1981). The community reaction increased the difficulty of trying to determine why so many people had high mercury levels, because repeat tests reflected the cessation of consumption by showing levels dropping dramatically from the time the first tests were reported. It was only by working with the community and gaining their trust that together it was possible to determine a cause and then to reassure them that for most adults, it was not necessary to restrict consumption of most country foods. However, it was recommended that care should be taken with seal liver, beluga and lake trout, and pregnant women should try to avoid eating these species or consume them in small quantities if other foods were available (Wheatley and Wheatley, 1981). This incident showed how poor, inaccurate and misleading information can exacerbate a problem which is already difficult to understand and is perceived as a threat.

AKWESASNE

Akwesasne, meaning "land where the partridge drums", lies on the St. Lawrence River straddling the Canada-U.S. border, where Ontario and Quebec meet. "*Kaniatarowaneneh*" - the majestic and magnificent river - was the focal point of all activity for the Mohawks, providing trade routes, food, and water for crops and livestock. The St. Lawrence became the site of a major construction project in the 1950s. The construction of the St. Lawrence Seaway, with its associated dams and power stations, had far-reaching consequences for the community. Much of the farm land was flooded and trees and wildlife habitats were destroyed. Cheap power increased industrial activity, including pulp and paper mills, which discharged toxic waste into the air and water, affecting both farming and fishing. With fish contaminated by mercury and other chemicals, people were afraid to eat it. Where there had been 104 commercial fishermen prior to construction, there were only 11 by 1990 (F. Henry Lickers, Director, Environment Division, Mohawk Council of Akwesasne, personal communication). With traditional foods contaminated, alternative foods were sought. Change in diet, from high protein fish and meat to high carbohydrate "junk" foods, and associated change in lifestyle, contributed to a prevalence of diabetes four times the Canadian average (Wheatley, B. 1994) where there had been none fifty years earlier.

Much of the traditional culture revolved around the production, harvesting and sharing of food. When these activities are no longer possible, the impact is considerable. A formerly proud, self-sufficient, healthy population now has about 44% of the population unemployed, receiving social assistance. The breakdown in traditional roles and relationships associated with traditional lifestyles and consequent loss of control over many aspects of life has contributed to problems of drug and alcohol abuse, and violence associated with gambling and smuggling in the community (Johansen, 1993). Akwesasne thus illustrates how environmental contaminants, including mercury, have disrupted the harmonious balance which was central to the traditional culture and lifestyle, with resulting negative effects on health and well being.

5. Discussion

Degradation of the environment by western industrial development, including by contaminants such as mercury, is seen by Aboriginal people as lack of respect. The harmonious balance on which Aboriginal people's philosophy is based has been disrupted by forces outside their control. The ability to provide for present and future generations, an integral part of this philosophy, is threatened. The knowledge that traditional foods contain mercury may produce a range of social and cultural impacts, apart from any direct health effects. Concern about these foods may result in change in diet, replacing high protein traditional foods with affordable alternatives, which is difficult in remote or northern communities (Wheatley, M.A., 1994). High carbohydrate foods are usually least expensive. In addition, serious social problems may result from the inability to follow traditional lifestyles which were integrative social activities affording the opportunity to learn skills and values. The loss of both the subsistence and economic base removes the ability to be a good provider for the family and the community, a highly valued trait. The new lifestyle is often less active and less social and this contributes to family and community violence, drug and alcohol abuse and suicide or attempted suicide. Also, change in diet and lifestyle contributes to loss of fitness (Rode and Shephard, 1994) and chronic disease conditions such and diabetes, at the same time that the social and cultural benefits of harvesting and eating traditional foods are being lost. These impacts are reinforced by perceptions of risk and reality which are influenced by holistic concepts of environment and health and further exacerbated by problems of communication. For Aboriginal people, taking action to restore or rehabilitate the environment is an essential step in the healing of both individuals and communities.

References

Berger, T.R.: 1977, *Northern Frontier, Northern Homeland.* (2 vols). Supply and Services Canada, Ottawa.

Erikson, K.: 1994, *A New Species of Trouble: Explorations of Disaster, Trauma, and Community.* W.W. Norton and Company, New York.

Guttormson, K.: 1995, Whitedog fights use of thinner by natives. *Victoria Times-Colonist*, May 26, 1995, p. A17 (originally published in *Winnipeg Free Press*).

James Bay and Northern Quebec Native Harvesting Research Committee: 1979, *Research to establish present levels of native harvesting. Harvest by the Inuit of Northern Quebec. Phase II (Yr. 1976).* Montreal,.

Johansen, B.E.: 1993, *Life and death in Mohawk country.* Fulcrum Publishing, Golden, CO.

McClellan, C.: 1987, *Part of the Land, Part of the Water.* Douglas and McIntyre Ltd., Vancouver.

Rode, A. and Shephard, R.J.: 1994, Acculturation and loss of fitness in the Inuit. The preventive role of active leisure. *Arct. Med. Res.* 53, Suppl. 2, 213-217

Shkilnyk, A.M.: 1985, *A Poison Stronger than Love: The Destruction of an Ojibwa Community.* Yale University Press, New Haven.

Slovic, P., Fischhoff, B. and Lichtenstein, S.: 1982, Risk perception. Facts versus fears: Understanding perceived risk. In D. Kahneman and P. Slovic, (Eds.) *Judgment under uncertainties. Heuristics and biases.* Cambridge University Press, New York, 463-489.

Wheatley, B.: 1995, Exposure of Aboriginal peoples in Canada to methylmercury with an emphasis on the Northwest Territories. *Proceedings of the workshop "Mercury-A health concern in the NWT".* Dept. of Health and Social Services, GNWT, Yellowknife.

Wheatley, B.: 1994, A new approach to assessing the effects of environmental contaminants on Aboriginal peoples. *Arct. Med. Res.*. 53, Suppl. 2, 386-390.

Wheatley, B. and Paradis, S.: 1995, Exposure of Canadian Aboriginal Peoples to methylmercury. *Water, Air and Soil Pollution* 80,5-11

Wheatley, M.A.: 1996, The importance of social and cultural effects of mercury on Aboriginal peoples. *NeuroTox.* 17(1), 251-256.

Wheatley, M.A.: 1995, The social and cultural effects of environmental contaminants on Aboriginal peoples. *Proceedings of the workshop "Mercury - A health concern in the NWT".* Dept. of Health and Social Services, GNWT, Yellowknife.

Wheatley, M.A.: 1994, Aboriginal health and the environment. *Arct. Med. Res.* 53, Suppl. 2, 265-267.

Wheatley, M.A. and Wheatley, B.: 1981, The effect of eating habits on mercury levels among Inuit residents of Sugluk, P.Q. *Études/Inuit/Studies.* 5(1), 27-43.

RISK ASSESSMENT OF MERCURY IN ALTA FLORESTA. AMAZON BASIN - BRAZIL

S. HACON*, E. R ROCHEDO*, R. CAMPOS** , G. ROSALES**, L. D. LACERDA ***
*IRD/CNEN, **PUC-RJ,*** UFF
* Instituto de Radioproteção e Dosimetria - Av. Salvador Allende s/n - Cx. Postal 37750 - Jacarepaguá - Rio de Janeiro - Brasil.

ABSTRACT. In the last 15 years gold mining activity has been the main source of the mercury (Hg) emissions into the atmosphere in the Amazon Basin. The first phase of gold production takes place in remote areas. In general the second one happens in the local urban area, where the gold is commercialized and sent to the great economic centers. In the last 3 years, this activity started to decline as a consequence of the high cost of the gold production but in the Municipality of Alta Floresta, the gold trade still plays an important role in the local economy.This paper addresses the assessment of the Hg exposure scenarios and their quantitative risk for inhalation of metallic Hg vapor and for ingestion of total Hg, using indirect exposure measurements, for different age groups of the urban area of Alta Floresta. This work took into account the field study which provided background information, such as characteristics of local and regional environment, Hg concentrations in different environmental media, and the character of the local urban population. The mean levels of Hg in the atmosphere of the urban area ranged from 210 ng/m^3 to 880 ng/m^3. Alta Floresta has no riverside population and there is a low fish consumption rate of 8 g/d among the general population. However, mercury levels in locally consumed carnivorous fish, ranged from 0.3 to 3.6 mg/kg, depending on the species and on the period of the year. The levels of mercury in soil surrounding the residential areas near the Hg emissions sources, ranged from 0.05 to 4.10 mg/kg. Hg in soil may represent an important source of mercury ingestion for local children up to 4 years of age. The mean Hazard Index estimated for the general adult population was 1.4. For the general population, regarding the number of persons exposed in the urban area, inhalation of metallic Hg vapor is the main route of exposure. The results for water ingestion for all groups are negligible. For families of fishermen the Hazard Index was estimated to be 9.3, with a contribution of 92% from fish ingestion.

1. Introduction

In the Amazon, metallic mercury has been widely used in gold production by the informal mining sector known as "garimpos". Since the late seventies, gold has been extracted from soil or river sediments through amalgamation with mercury; the amalgam is then heated, giving off mercury vapors while leaving the ore. This Hg has the potential to contaminate the environment, being transported long distances before being deposited on the earth's surface and entering the aquatic food chain. The second phase of gold production occurs in urban areas, where the gold trading takes place. The gold from garimpos has some impurities of which Hg accounts for 2 to 8%. The amalgamated gold is repeatedly burnt to completely separate the two components, until reaching pure gold. From 1980 until 1994 the gold trade in the urban area of Alta Floresta had an estimated production ranging from 1 to 2 tons of gold per month (Hacon *et al*, 1995). The Hg vapor is emitted directly into the urban atmosphere, where a population of about 46,000 inhabitants has been potentially exposed to Hg emissions during the last 15 years.

The health risk assessment of Hg should approach the regional, local and multimedia aspects of Hg fate and transport in this environment. Alta Floresta is a municipality in the state of Mato Grosso in the Amazon Basin, 800 km away from Cuiabá, capital of the state. It is not a riverside area but the Teles Pires River, 67 km from the urban area, is a main fishing resource for the region, with an important role for the local economy due to the intensive gold mining activity established in the decade of the 80's. Teles Pires River contributes about 80% of the fish consumed by the local population of Alta Floresta. Mercury deposited into water bodies is transformed into methylmercury (MeHg) through the activity of bacteria present in soil, sediments and suspended particulates in water. Organic mercury gets into the trophic chains where it can be biomagnified a million fold between initial transformation and the ultimate predatory species, mainly fish. Recent findings indicate that MeHg levels in carnivorous fish from Alta Floresta rivers accounts for 85% to 100% of total Hg (Akagi *et al*, 1993). The largest predatory fishes from Amazon rivers present the highest MeHg levels. However, the fish consumption pattern for the general population of Alta Floresta is low, which makes this local scenario different from that for the riverside population.

The population of Alta Floresta is exposed to organic and inorganic compounds via different pathways. Exposure and effects of toxic substances depend on various factors: levels of contamination in the medium, the existence of potential pathways for human exposure, the size and nature of the community likely to be exposed and the duration and magnitude of the exposure. The great majority of the inhabitants of Alta Floresta has different social and cultural characteristics than other Amazon communities (Boischio *et al,* 1995, Hacon, 1996). This fact is important in understanding why Alta Floresta has a different exposure scenario in relation to other "garimpo" areas.

2 STUDY AREA AND METHODS

The present study has been carried out in the urban area of Alta Floresta, in the Southern part of Amazon Basin. The region started to be occupied in the decade of the 70's by a private colonization project, which had the aim of developing a large scale agricultural project. However, the "gold rush" in the early's 80 in the Amazon Basin transformed the original social-economic project for the region into an important gold trade center. About 70% of the population came from south and southeast of Brazil with social and cultural habits different from the indigenous amazonian population. The main economic activity of this region is the gold trade, which until 1994, was responsible for an average emission factor of Hg for the atmosphere, ranging from 0.5 and 2.5 tons of per year (Hacon *et al,* 1995). The variation of the Hg emissions depends on variables such as the type of technology of the "garimpo", the amount of Hg amalgamated by kg of gold, the total amount of gold trade and the current price of gold. Those people from the gold shops are primarily exposed to Hg emissions at the workplace and also in the urban environment. For the general population, the Hg from the urban atmosphere is the main source of exposure. Hg contamination has been studied at the workplaces and the environment of the region of Alta floresta since 1990 (CETEM 1992; Hacon *et al*, 1993; 1995; Hacon, 1996). These studies provided background information, such as the characteristics of Hg sources and Hg concentrations in different environmental media, physical, social and economic characteristics of local and regional environment. People in Alta Floresta, as well as many other areas of Amazon Basin, have been exhaustively studied and used as information sources for Hg exposure studies but it has been difficult to get biological samples from them. Through the present methodology, one is able to simulate the potential health risk, identifying the spot groups that should be of the greatest concern.

2.1 Characterization of the population

In 1992, a survey about the concern of Hg contamination in the urban area was carried out among the residents, gold trade dealers and local governments. In 1993, as result of this survey, an extension of 50 km^2 of the urban area, which concentrates about 70% of the urban population and all gold dealers shops were integrated into the present study in order to evaluate Hg exposures. The next step was to assess a sample of the population that could simulate the various groups related to Hg exposure in the urban area. A sample of 160 adult inhabitants from a random list have been interviewed during the dry season (May to September). About 50% of the interviewed individuals were from the local trading and the other 50% from homes, between 15 and 60 years old and from both sexes. A questionnaire was applied in order to get demographic, anthropometric measures (weight and height), socio-economic and occupational activities information, and dietary habits, with emphasis on fish preferences and consumption (Hacon, 1996). To estimate the amount of fish ingested we have weighted the amount of fish to be consumed in the next meal in 10 % of households. The information about the groups under 15 years old was obtained from interviews with their parents. The information drawn from this survey was fundamental to identifying potential exposure pathways for Hg and to define the exposed groups.

Occupational exposure in this study includes individuals from both sexes who work in the gold trade activity who are directly and indirectly exposed to metallic Hg vapor emissions due to the amalgam burning. The exposure in the workplaces (gold shops) is intermittent, with the higher concentrations occuring during the burning time. When the shops have a reasonable exhausting system, a large part of the Hg emissions goes to the external atmosphere. Otherwise, most of it remains indoors and it gets dispersed through the doors and windows.

2.2 Environmental Contamination

A multimedia approach to the environmental monitoring program for Hg was carried out, taking into account the Hg emission sources and the main Hg contamination pathways for the urban population of Alta Floresta (Hacon, 1996). Mercury is present in the atmosphere in particulate and gaseous phases and in various chemical forms. In Alta Floresta metallic mercury vapor (Hg^0) accounts for about 90% of the total Hg in the atmosphere. Hg measurement programs were established for water, fish, and for outdoor and indoor air, the later inside the gold trade shops. Secondary data has been used to estimate the exposure due to soil ingestion. The soil ingestion rate for children was obtained from the literature and personal judgement (Hacon, 1996). This program was carried out during the dry season because it is the worst period in terms of air quality, due to the intensity of the "garimpo" activity, which coincides with the biomass burn period. Three sites were set up for air Hg samples in the urban area. The location of the stations took into account meteorological parameters, sources of Hg emissions and residential and work places. Gaspar station, in the central area of the city, is close to the majority of gold dealers shops. Airport station is upwind and Boa Nova station is downwind relative to the predominant wind direction.

The initial aim, in relation to the indoor Hg sampling program, was to use individual sampler systems to evaluate the workers Hg exposure during the time of amalgam burning but this was not possible due to the internal conditions of the gold shop and the lack of permission from the gold dealers to use the samplers only during the burning period (Hacon, 1996). Thus, our option was to evaluate the Hg exposure indoor through the average exposure at the workplace. Four gold shops were chosen for this assessment, taking into account internal burning conditions, number of workers and the amount of gold commercialized weekly (>10 kg/week) (Hacon *et al*, 1995). Total Atmospheric Hg was sampled in two successive bubble traps containing 5% KMnO4 in sulfuric acid 2N. The flow-rate of about 1 liter per minute was controlled by rotameter. The same sampling system was used for indoor and environmental samples.Trapping efficiency was better than 90%. Inside the gold shops, we assume that the exposure to Hg is 100% in vapor phase, estimated using the 90% percentile indoor Hg concentration distribution (X90%). This approach was chosen considering the distance from the amalgam burning place inside the shops and the location of the sampling system used, in order to have a better evaluation of the workers's exposure. The indoor Hg exposure levels ranged from 70 to 40 600 $\mu g/m^3$. This range is dependent on the season and the amount of amalgam burnt daily (Hacon, 1996).

The inhalation rate varies with age, sex, and physical activities. The average value for inhalation rate used for adults and children is 20 m^3/d and 10 m^3/d, respectively (EPA, 1989 b). We assume the same inhalation rate value for gold shop workers as that for the general public, because their activity does not require physical effort, corrected for the estimated exposure time. We also assumed 100% of absorption of Hg by the lungs.

The water bodies and wells used for water supply were sampled using a acid solution of

$K_2Cr_2O_7$ at 0,01% and HNO_3 at 5% (Campos *et al*, 1990). The different fish species were weighed and immediately frozen (Hacon *et al*, 1993). The mercury analysis was performed by cold vapor atomic absorption spectrometry (CVAAS) after wet digestion. The gold trap technique has been used for measurements of Hg in water. The detection limit for total Hg was of 10 ng/m^3 for air, 0,3 ng/l for water and 0.1 µg/kg (w.w) for fish (Campos *et al*, 1990). Analytical quality was assured by several methods such as a blank control (3 blanks for a batch of 10 samples), duplicate analysis and the analysis of reference materials with the Interlaboratory Comparison Program, Ottawa, Canada.

2.3 Exposure Assessment

Probabilistic calculation was used to evaluate the urban population exposure and to estimate the risks for different groups of the population. The parameters used as input for the modelling are presented in Table 1. The Hg dose rate was estimated for different routes and variable values dependant on site conditions and/or the characteristics of the potentially exposed population group. The general equations for assessment of chronic exposure for ingestion and inhalation were applied (EPA, 1989a):

a) Ingestion intake.

$$I_{ing}\ (mg/(kg.d)) = \frac{IC\ .\ IR}{BW} \qquad (1)$$

where: IC = Fish or soil Hg concentration (mg/kg) or water (ng/l)
IR = Ingestion Rate, (kg_{FISH} / meal, l_{water}/day, kg_{soil}/day)
BW = Body weight, (kg)

b) Inhalation intake.

$$I_{air}(mg/(kg.d)) = \frac{CA\ .\ IR}{BW} \qquad (2)$$

where: CA = Hg concentration in air, (mg/m^3)
IR = inhalation rate, (m^3/d)
BW = Body weight, (kg)

c) Potential health risk.
The hazard quotient (HQ) is calculated as the dimensionless ratio of the estimated dose rate, I, to the selected reference dose (RfD) µg/kg/day:

$$HQ = \frac{I}{RfD} \qquad (3)$$

If HQ is less than one, there is no anticipated risk for adverse health effects. If HQ is equal to or greater than one, there is a possibility for adverse health effects to occur for sensitive population groups. For risk assessment purposes it is better if one can determine a Reference Dose (RfD) which is protective even for the most sensitive groups of the population. The oral RfD for both inorganic and methyl mercury is 0.3 μg/kg/d b.w (Young, 1992). There is no reference dose for inhalation. The usual way is to use the reference concentration for inhalation (RfC) 0,3 μg/m³ (IRIS, 1993) however, even knowing that organic and inorganic Hg pose different risks, we assume the same RfD value (0.3 μg/kg/d) to simulate the inhalation and ingestion exposure and to estimate the potential risk. Although recognizing that different exposure routes can lead to different risk end points, in this work for the comparison of relative relevances, all doses have been summed to get a combined hazard quotient for each studied group.

Table 1-Values of the input parameters for the Risk Assessment Modelling.

parameters	unit	distrib.	mean	s.d
[Hg] water	ng/l	ln	3,0	1.8
[Hg] Fish	μg/kg	n	1320	737
[Hg] environmental air	μg/m³	ln	0.5	0.92
[Hg] indoors air	μg/m³	ln	26.2	2.82
[Hg] Soil	mg/kg	ln	0.23	0.02
water ingestion rate (adult)	l/d	t	2.0	-
water ingestion rate (children)	l/d	t	1.0	-
fish ingestion rate - Group 1 e 3	kg/d	ln	0.008	0.006
fish ingestion rate - Group 5	kg/d	ln	0.005	0.006
fish ingestion rate - Group 4	kg/d	ln	0.005	0.006
fish ingestion rate - Group 2	kg/d	ln	0.110	0.045
fish ingestion rate - Group 6	kg/d	ln	0.080	0.025
soil ingestion rate - Group 4	kg/d	ln	0.005	0.025
workers's inhalation rate	m³/d	t	10	-
inhalation rate for general	m³/d	t	20	-
inhalation rate for children-	m³/d	t	10	
body weight - adult population	kg	t	60	-
body weight - workers	Kg	t	65	
body weight - children (5- 14)	Kg	t	32	
body weight - chidren (1- 4)	kg	t	15	
RfD total Hg	μg/kg/d	lu	0.3	-

ln = lognormal lu= log uniform t= triangular

2.4 Uncertainty Analyses

Probabilistic calculations were performed for the quantitative uncertainty analysis by Monte Carlo simulation, using the Crystal Ball software (Decisioneering, 1993). The Latin Hypercube Sampling method was used with 1000 iterations to define the probabilistic distribution of the variables and identify the parameters that could significantly contribute to the uncertainty on model predictions (Gardner, 1988; Rochedo, 1994). For the uncertainty analysis, each parameter is associated with a distribution described by a mean value, a standard deviation and maximum and minimum values. These values are those most representative of the assumed distribution (e.g., arithmetic mean for a normal distribution and geometric mean for a lognormal distribution). The distributions have been chosen according to state of art scientific evidence and personal considerations about the studied scenarios.

3 - Results and Discussion

The baseline exposure scenario for the urban population of Alta Floresta is a low level chronic exposure. This scenario includes different exposure pathways for both adults and children populations. The groups were characterized in function of their pattern of exposure, fish consumption habits, activities and age:

For adults - Group 1- The general population
Group 2- the fishermen's families
Group 3- workers from the gold shops.

For children - Group 4- children from general population (1-4 years old)
Group 5-children from the general population (5-14 years old)
Group 6- fishermen's children (5-14 years old).

3.1 Characterization of the urban population

The age range from 15 to 34 years old, represents 68% of the sample population and also represents the range of age of the economically active. This feature may be explained by the colonization process of the region in the early 80's (Hacon, 1996). In relation to the occupational activity, 34% of the women, between 17 to 39 years old, mentioned having worked in the "garimpos" activity, as cookers. All of them, reported having suffered from malaria, which is seen as a confounding variable relative to the symptoms of Hg contamination. Nowadays, they are household workers and are not directly exposed to metallic Hg vapor emissions. However, they are still exposed to secondary levels, from the urban environment atmosphere. 30% have been working in the urban area, close to the gold shops, as sellers in commercial activities or in administration. 36% are household workers and have never worked out. For men, 70% reported to have worked in "garimpo" activity, of which 44.5% burnt amalgam at least part of the time during 5 years. In relation to sanitary conditions, 82 % of the adults interviewed use water from wells, without any type of primary treatment, and about 16% use water from a supply system.

3.2 Exposure Assessment

The exposure level for a standard water consumption of 2 l/d for the adult population was estimated to be 0.1 ng/kg/d. This exposure route can be regarded as negligible.

The levels of Hg in carnivorous fish are high, ranging from 0.3 to 3.6 mg/kg (w.w), as in many other areas of the Amazon Basin (Akagi *et al*, 1993; Malm *et al*, 1990; Aula *et al*, 1995). About 95% of the fish consumed by the urban group are carnivorous fish. The highest Hg concentrations were found in *Brachyplastystoma spp* (Piraiba), that accounts for 29% of local consumption. The Hg concentration in this specie ranged from 1.7 to 3.6 mg/kg. The most consumed species is the *Paulicea Lutkeni* (Jau), accounting for about 33% of local consumption and has Hg concentrations ranging from 0.4 to 2.7 mg/kg. The carnivorous species that have an average Hg level greater than 0.5 mg/kg make up 80% of the total consumption (Hacon *et al*, 1993). The daily intake of Hg for the urban population was estimated assuming a weighted average fish concentration of 1.3 mg/kg (Hacon, 1996). About 10% of the urban population interviewed does not eat any type of fish. The fishermen (group 2) are the people with the highest average fish ingestion rates (110 g/d). Groups 1 and 3 presented the same average fish ingestion rate of 8 g/. Group 4 (children, 1-4 years old) has an average rate ingestion of the 5 g/d. The statistic F-test showed that there is not a significant difference between the fish ingestion rate for all children in this age range. The highest fish consumption was verified in group 6, fishermen's children, above 5 years old, with a mean ingestion rate of 80 g/d. The body weights for the different groups were used to correct the estimated total daily Hg dose.

In play-grounds close to the gold shops, Hg concentration reaches values up to 9 $\mu g/m^3$ in air and 4 mg/kg in soils. The Hg in soils is due to the deposition process, and can vary as a function of the Hg rate emission, the distance from the source and meteorological parameters. The soil exposure was estimated for group 4 (children below 5 years), due to their exhibited mouthing behavior, because soil and dust particles were observed on their hands during normal playing activities, and also due to the proximity of the residential and school areas to the gold shops.

We assume the same mean exposure levels of metallic Hg vapor, 0.5 $\mu g/m^3$, for all of the urban population, that comprises people resident or workers of the urban area, although the air concentrations measured ranged from < 0.02 to 5.8 $\mu g/m^3$. Only for the workers from the gold shops, were different exposure patterns regarded. These workers are exposed about 10 hours per day to high Hg levels (mean 26.2 $\mu g/m^3$) and the rest of the time they are exposed to the same environmental concentrations as the general population. The women workers from the gold shops, in general do not burn amalgamam directly, because they work in administrative tasks. However, due to cultural habits, they stay indoors all the time while men usually go out very often to drink or to talk.

Table 2 shows the results for mean dose and hazard quotients (HQ) for the different exposure pathways, with a confidence level of 95%. Group 1, the general urban population, would be unlikely to experience adverse health effects due to all pathways. However, the maximum HQ values for ingestion (18.3) and inhalation (9.5) show that there may be individuals with critical values which should be better investigated. For group 2, fishermen's families, the fish ingestion is the main exposure pathway, with an Hg daily intake of 2.23 μg/kg bw, which is about 7.5 times higher than the reference dose. This exposure pathway contributes 92% to the hazard index. The HQ for this group (8.6) is a value of concern, mainly for pregnant women as it is known that Hg may reach the fetus with health consequences for the child. The maximum HQ value for this group (76.5) indicates that some individuals, mainly the more sensitive ones, have a great probability of exihibiting adverse health effects.

Group 3, the gold shops's workers, presented a mean inhalation dose estimated at 4.5 μg/kg/d, equivalent to a HQ of 9.21 The maximum value for HQ (48.2) indicates the probability of critical sub-groups. Even being intermittent, the Hg exposure can be characterized as a chronic exposure, taking into account the time, magnitude and duration of the exposure. Comparing the average exposure levels (26.2 $\mu g/m^3$) with the threshold limit value (TLV) for Hg vapor in the workplace (50 $\mu g/m^3$), the Hg exposure levels in the gold shops are below the threshold, despite the fact they have a long-term (8 years) exposure. Nevertheless, it is the frequent complaint of workers that they have symptoms that can be attributed to Hg intoxication (tremor, erethism, paresthesia, insomnia, lack of self-control, weakness, renal alteration). It is difficult to associate these to Hg exposure due to the presence of confounding variables, caused by parasitic, infection, endemic, and other diseases. However, the highest value from the hazard quotient (48.2) may be strongly correlated with these symptoms.

For group 4, children between 1-4 year old, inhalation of Hg vapor contributes 36.4%, fish 45.4% and soil ingestion 18%, for the total dose. The total daily dose for this group is 1.1μg/kg/ bw, 3.6 times higher than the total Hg RfD of 0.3 μg/kg bw. The probabilistic values for the maximum inhalation and ingestion HQ show the possibility of the existence of critical sub-groups which have to be better investigated. Taking into account that this group was exposed since the pregnancy stage, they should be followed-up and studied in terms of dose-response relationship.

For group 5, the general urban population's children from 5 to 14 years old, , the main exposure pathway is inhalation from the urban air, with a contribution of 72%, while the ingestion of fish contributes 28% to the total dose. The maximum value for this group also confirms the importance of the inhalation route, with a HQ of 22.5. Group 5 has an average low fish ingestion rate and consequently a low HQ for ingestion. However, the individuals with the highest ingestion rate, 50g/d, showed HQ of 6.2 for this route of exposure.

Table 2 - Risk Assessment For The Different Groups of the Population

Groups	Routes of Exposure	Medium	dose µg/kg/d	Hazard Quotient (HQ)		
				mean	max.	distr.
Group 1	ingestion	water	0.0001	0.0003	0.002	ln
		fish	0.2	0.7	18.3	ln
	inhalation	air	0.2	0.7	9.5	ln
	Hazard Index		0.41	1.43	28.0	
Group 2	ingestion	water	0.0001	0.0003	0.002	ln
		fish	2.23	8.60	76.5	ln
	inhalation	air	0.2	0.7	9.5	ln
	Hazard Index		2.44	9.33	86.2	
Group 3	ingestion	water	0.0001	0.0003	0.002	ln
		fish	0.2	0.7	18.3	ln
	inhalation	air	4.50	9.21	48.2	ln
	Hazard Index		4.70	9.93	66.7	
Group 4	ingestion	water	0.0002	0.07	0.3	Ln
		soil	0.2	0.5	2.0	Ln
		fish	0.5	1.4	9.2	Ln
	inhalation	air	1.0	3.5	11.7	Ln
	Hazard Index		1.72	5.47	23.2	
Group 5	ingestion	water	0.0001	0.03	0.3	Ln
		fish	0.2	0.9	6.2	Ln
	inhalation	air	0.5	1.5	22.5	Ln
	Hazard Index		0.70	2.43	29.0	
Grupo 6	ingestion	water	0.0001	0.03	0.3	Ln
		fish	3.50	8.82	75.0	Ln
	inhalation	air	0.5	1.5	22.5	Ln
	Hazard Index		4.0	10.4	98.0	

For group 6, fishermen's children, fish ingestion is the main exposure pathway with a mean Hg daily dose of 3.5 μg/kg bw. This value is above the LOAEL (lowest-observed-adverse-effect level, 3 μg/kg bw), recognized as the lower limit for paraesthesia symptoms. This exposure route contributes about 85% for the Hazard Index. The probabilistic maximum HQ values for this exposure is 75, confirming the existence of critical sub-groups in the children's population. This study shows a moderate fish consumption by the urban population of Alta Floresta. However, one has to take into account that even with about half the ingestion rate in relation to the riverside population (200g/d) (Boischio *et al*, 1995), the levels of Hg in carnivorous fish from the Teles Pires River are a threat to this group of the population.

3.3 Uncertainty Analysis

The use of the quantitative uncertainty analysis allowed the determination of the most sensitive parameters in the overall uncertainty assessment of risk. This analysis is an important tool for decision making, providing information that could not be obtained from the standard point estimate approach, and giving guidance to which parameters one must focus ones research studies on, since a better knowledge of actual values will lead to a reduction of uncertainty of risk estimates (Rochedo, 1994).

The uncertainty charts (Figures 1 and 2) show the probabilistic results for the contribution to the uncertainty of individual hazard quotient for each group studied and Table 3 presents the uncertainty contribution associated with each exposure route to the Hazard Index.

The uncertainty chart (Fig 1) shows that, for group 1, inhalation and fish ingestion have about the same contribution to the variability of the Hazard Index. The parameters of ingestion rate and Hg concentration in the urban atmosphere, dominate the uncertainty with a contribution of 72.3% and 94% to the variance, respectively, as presented in Table 3. For group 2, the Hazard Quotient is 9.3. The ingestion of fish is the route that dominates the variability of the Hazard Index, being the ingestion rate parameter with the greatest contribution for the variance. Hg concentrations in the atmosphere, even presenting the highest contribution for the variance (94%), does not have a great effect on the variability of model predictions. For group 3, the inhalation route dominates the variability of the model, being the Hg concentration at workplace parameter with the great contribution for the variance (97%). Some of this uncertainty is unavoidable however, because there are some factors interfering with this variable, such as microambient conditions, amount of amalgam burnt daily, sampling location, among others, which can be better investigated. Water ingestion does not contribute significantly for any group exposed to Hg.

We regarded a static model for the children exposure. However, we know that for this population group, age is an important factor of variability associated with habits. The hazard index for groups 4 and 5 were estimated in 5.5 and 2.4 respectively. The soil ingestion pathway, is not so important when compared with fish ingestion and air inhalation. The uncertainty chart (Fig 2) shows for groups 4 and 5 that the HQ for inhalation is the main contribution to the variability of the Hazard Index and the Hg concentration in the urban atmosphere dominates the uncertainty, with a contribution of 90% and 95% to the variance, respectively. This variability is due to the large range of Hg concentrations in the urban atmosphere from 10 μg/m3 to 5400 μg/m3, which varies with the amount of Hg emitted daily to the atmosphere, meteorological parameters and distance from the residences to the emission sources. For group 6 (fishermen families's children) the hazard index is 10. The fish ingestion is the route that dominates the variability of the hazard index, being the ingestion rate parameter that contributes with 59% for the variance. Hg concentrations in air also have some contribution to the variance.

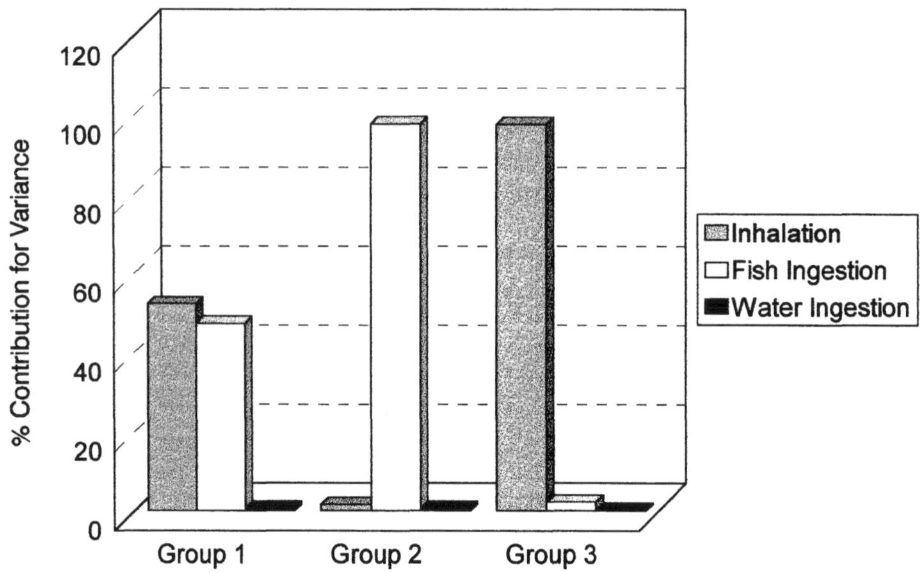

Figure 1 - Uncertainty Analysis for Adult Population Scenarios

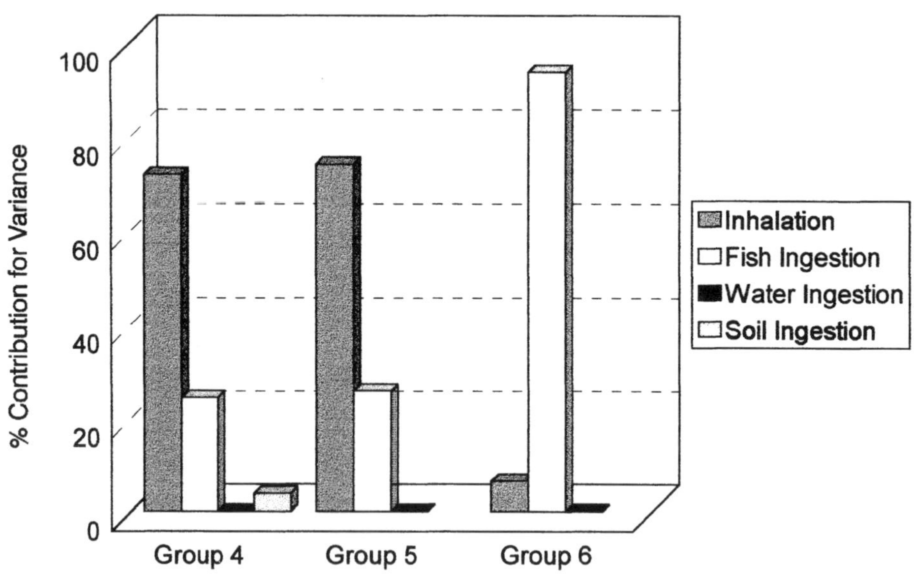

Figure 2 - Uncertainty Analysis for Children Population Scenarios

Table 3 - Uncertainty Analyis for the Exposure Scenario

Groups	Route exposure	Medium	Contribution for the variance (%)			
			[Hg]	Rates	B.W	RfD
Group 1	Ingestion	water	77.5	-	4.5	17.8
		fish	20.0	72.3	2.0	5.0
	Inhalation	air	94.0	0.2	2.0	3.8
Group 2	Ingestion	water	77.5	-	4.5	17.8
		fish	28.5	52.0	3.0	16.5
	Inhalation	air	94.0	0.2	2.0	3.8
Group 3	Ingestion	water	77.5	-	4.5	18.0
		fish	20.0	72.3	2.0	5.0
	Inhalation	air	97.0	1.5	1.5	-
Group 4	Ingestion	water	93	-	7	-
		fish	49	30	10	11
		soil	7	18	30	45
	Inhalation	air	90	0.5	3.5	6
Group 5	Ingestion	water	96	2	2	-
		fish	44	37	5	14
	Inhalation	air	95	-	0.5	4.5
Group 6	ingestion	water	96	2	2	-
		fish	27	59	1.5	12
	inhalation	air	95	-	0.5	4.5

4- Conclusion

The baseline exposure scenario for the general urban population of Alta Floresta is the low level chronic exposure. However, the health risk assessment methodology allowed the identification of spot groups, who can be regarded as risk groups for each exposure pathway. In relation to workers, a great deal of the information on effects associated with inhalation exposure to Hg vapor comes from studies conducted with occupational workers. However, in Alta Floresta, the gold shop workers can not be compared with the traditional mining or industrial workers, as they have different exposure patterns, professional behavior and habits, in relation to workers with a formal activity, where the work legislation is applied and enforced. Nevertheless, this is the group with the highest priority in terms of dose-response relationship. In relation to fish ingestion, the women from the fishermen's families are the spot group. Not only them but also their children should be followed up,on in terms of neurological damage.

In relation to the children's population, the health risk groups, with the maximum HQ value, should have a great priority, because there is evidence that children may be more susceptible to Hg toxicity because of increased absorption and retention of Hg and the high sensitivity of their developing nervous system. In addition, some children are hypersensitive to mercury exposure.

In Alta Floresta during the dry season we observed a high incidence of respiratory diseases. However, this can also be associated with the period of biomass burning, when the levels of particulate material increases to 25 times higher than that during the rainy season. Nevertheless, it is difficult to determine whether effects observed in the exposed population are directly attributable to Hg exposure due to the presence of multiple confounding variables, such as malnutrition, parasitic, infectious and endemic diseases (malaria), poor health care and lack of information on Hg intoxication among local doctors. The difficulties are associated with the non- specific nature of individual symptoms, and the lack of a clear diagnostic criteria for low-dose Hg intoxication.

ACKNOWLEDGMENTS

The authors would like to thank to Luiz Tadeu Duarte from IRD, for the support on computing; Dra. Lilian P. de Moraes, for application of the questionnaires, and Saturnino J.S. Filho, from the Secretaria de Saúde de Alta Floresta, for the support on infrastructure in the Hg sampling program; Dr. C. Tobar and Dr. P. Artaxo for the incentive and financial support; and, to the institutions FINEP/PADCT, FIOCRUZ, CNPq and CAPES, which also contributed with financial support.

REFERENCES

AKagi, H., Malm, O., Kinjo, Y., Harada, M., Branches, F., *et al.*: 1993, In: Proc. of the International Symposium on Assessment of Environmental Pollution and Health Effects from Methylmercury, Kumamoto, Japan, 41-48.

Aula, I., Braunschweiler, H., Leino, T., Malim, I., Porvari, P., *et al.*: 1995, In: Mercury Pollution, Integration and Synthesis. Watras, C. & Huckabee, J.W. (Eds). Lewis Publishers 21-40.

Boischio, A.A., Henshel, D., Barbosa, A.: 1995, Ecosystem Health. 1, 177-192.

Campos, R.C., & Curtis, A.J.: 1990, In: Riscos e Consequências do Uso de Mercúrio, Seminário Nacional, FINEP, Rio de Janeiro, 110-134.

CETEM: 1992 Diagnóstico Preliminar dos Impactos Ambientais Gerados por Garimpos de Ouro em Alta Floresta/MT. CETEM/CNPq. Rio de Janeiro, 190 pages.

Decisioneering: 1993, Crystal Ball Version 3.0- Decisioneering Inc., Colorado.

Environmental Protection Agency (EPA): 1989 aExposure Assessment, In: Risk Assessment Guidance for Superfund. 1: 50 pages OSWER Directive 9285.7-01a, Office of Emergency and Remedial Response.

Environmental Protection Agency (EPA): 1989 b, Exposure Factors Handbook EPA 600/8/89/043, 157 pages.

Gardner, R.H.:1988, IOMOVS Report, NIRP, Swedish National Institute of Radiation Protection, Stockholm, Sweden, 64 pages.

Hacon, S., Campos, R.C., Rochedo, E.R. (1993) In: International Symposium Perspectives for Environmental Geochemistry in Tropical Countries, Niteroi. 115-120.

Hacon, S., Artaxo, P, Campos, R C., *et al.*: 1995. Water, Air and Soil Pollution. **80**: 273-283.

Hacon, S, 1996. Avaliação de Risco Potencial para a Saúde Humana da Exposição ao Mercúrio na Area Urbana de Alta Floresta. MT-Bacia Amazônica- Brasil. PhD dissertation UFF, Rio de Janeiro, 172 pages.

Environmental Protection Agency - Office of Research and Development:1993, IRIS. Integrated Risk Information System (data base).

Malm, O., Pfeiffer, W.C., Souza, C.M.M.: 1990, .Ambio. **19**, 11-15.

Rochedo, E.R.R.: 1994. PARATI-Modelo para a avaliação da exposição radiológica em um ambiente urbano após uma contaminação radioativa. PhD dissertation, IBCCF - UFRJ, Rio de Janeiro, 126 pages.

Young, R.A.: 1992, Toxicity Summary for Mercury. Prepared by Oak Ridge Resevation Environmental Restoration Program. 19 pages

ESTIMATING RISKS FROM EXPOSURE TO METHYLMERCURY: APPLICATION TO FIRST NATIONS PEOPLE IN CANADA

SARA HOOVER, RYAN HILL and TOM WATSON

Triton Environmental Consultants, Ltd.
#120-13511 Commerce Parkway, Richmond, B.C., V6V 2L1, Canada

Abstract. We combined dose-response analyses with a probabilistic exposure assessment to estimate the risks to native Canadians who ingest methylmercury via fish consumption from natural lakes and a reservoir in British Columbia. Available dose-response data included multivariate measurements of central nervous system functioning in Iraqi children exposed to methylmercury prenatally. We applied the method of principal components to simplify the data structure. The first principal component described close to 80% of the variability in the data, making it a reasonable choice as an index. The relationship between mercury in maternal hair and the probability of an abnormal neurological effects index was modeled with the logistic and Weibull functions. The goodness-of-fit of the two models is discussed and the results compared to other published dose-response analyses. Exposure distributions were developed to represent methylmercury dose by using observed data on methylmercury contamination in the lakes and reservoir and reasonable assumptions about other key parameters such as fish consumption. We estimated risks to the target population using Monte Carlo simulation. Consumption of reasonable quantities of fish from these bodies of water does not pose a significant risk to the aboriginal population.

1. Introduction

The Nechako Reservoir, shown in Figure 1, was created by impoundment of the Nechako River in the early 1950's. Flooding of a terrestrial system results in increased levels of mercury in the aquatic system and a stimulation of mercury methylation by bacteria (Jackson, 1988). Fish in such systems tend to accumulate higher levels of methylmercury. Measurements in the Nechako Reservoir showed the levels of mercury in rainbow trout were only somewhat elevated over natural lakes in the area (Triton, 1991), consistent with the old age of the reservoir.

To quantify the potential human health effects of consuming rainbow trout from the Nechako Reservoir we carried out a probabilistic risk assessment. We selected two lakes in the area for comparison to the reservoir. Ogston Lake showed background levels of methylmercury in trout (Triton, 1992). Fish from Tezzeron Lake, which lies on a geologic formation rich in mercury, had methylmercury levels similar to the Nechako Reservoir (Triton, 1992). Children of native women were selected as the target population, because developmental neurotoxicity is the most sensitive endpoint for mercury and aboriginals are the population most likely to consume significant quantities of fish from the reservoir. Dose-response analyses of the Iraqi poisoning episode (Marsh *et al.*, 1987) were combined with estimated distributions for methylmercury dose to characterize risks. The risks associated with ingestion of Nechako Reservoir fish were compared with those associated with the lakes as well as the general population.

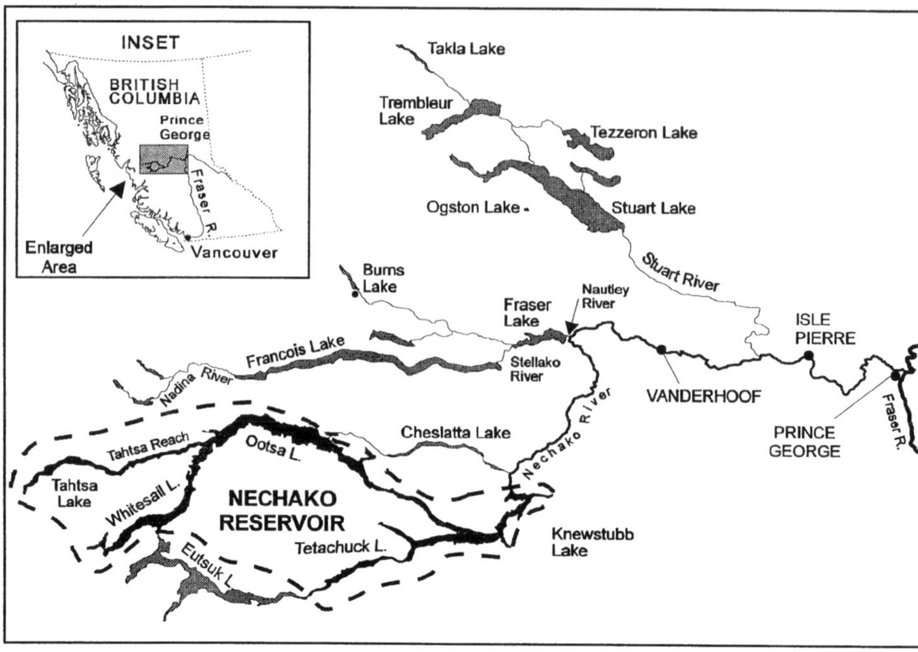

Figure 1. Map of Nechako Reservoir (indicated by dotted line) and surrounding area.

2. Analysis of Iraqi Dose-Response Data

Data from the Iraqi poisoning episode were used to relate neurological effects in infants to methylmercury dose. Marsh *et al.* (1987) estimated peak mercury levels in maternal hair during pregnancy, noted the presence or absence of symptoms such as paresthesia and seizures, and measured three quantitative variables related to neurologic functioning in the offspring. We applied principal components analysis to these multivariate data in order to construct a single index of neurologic effect. Principal components are linear combinations which reduce multivariate observations to a few summary variables (Selvin, 1995). The first principal component can often describe a significant percentage of the variance in the data, making it a useful summary index.

We selected the three quantitative variables of neurologic effect for principal components analysis: neurological score (CNS), age at first walking (Walk), and age at first talking (Talk). The computer program Stata® (Stata Corporation, 1993) was used to generate the coefficients for the principal components and the percent of variation explained by each component. The results are shown in Table 1. The first two principal components accounted for 94% of the variance in the data. The first principal component summarized close to 80% of the variation, making it a good index of neurologic effects. Data from Marsh *et al.* (1987) were used to select a cut-point between a "normal" (response variable equal to zero) and "abnormal" (response variable equal to one) value of the first principal component. As demonstrated in Table 1, the first principal component effectively identifies infants with two or more abnormal measures of neurologic functioning, as well as infants with an exceptionally high abnormal level in one of the three measures. The resulting quantal data set records peak maternal hair levels versus the occurrence of a normal or abnormal index value.

TABLE I
Results of principal components analysis

A. Variance accounted for by three principal components

Component	Variance	Proportion of variance explained	Cumulative proportion
1	2.32945	0.7765	0.7765
2	0.48737	0.1625	0.9389
3	0.18318	0.0611	1.0000

B. First principal component

$$P^{(1)} = 0.5427 \times \text{CNS} + 0.6154 \times \text{Walk} + 0.5716 \times \text{Talk}$$

C. Example calculations

	Normalized parameters				
	CNS	Walk	Talk	$P^{(1)}$ index	Response variable
Case 1	1.09	2.23[a]	1.90	3.05[b]	1
Case 2	2.19[a]	1.85[a]	1.71	3.30[b]	1
Case 3	0.73	1.11	2.28	2.38	0

[a] Abnormal values.
[b] Cut-off for abnormal $P^{(1)}$ index is 2.92.

The logistic model was fit to the dose-response data using maximum likelihood techniques (Hosmer and Lemeshow, 1989). A second analysis involved fitting the Weibull model (Morgan and Henrion, 1990) to the data. The functional forms of the two models are shown in Equations 1 and 2.

Logistic:

$$f(x) = \frac{1}{1 + e^{-(a+bx)}} \tag{1}$$

Weibull:

$$f(x) = 1 - e^{-\left(\frac{x}{c}\right)^k} \qquad (2)$$

To assess the fits of the two models, the Hosmer-Lemeshow X^2 (Hosmer and Lemeshow, 1989; Stata, 1993) was calculated. For this test the data were collapsed into 10 groups based on the percentiles of the predicted probabilities. The degrees of freedom are approximately equal to the number of groups minus 2, or 8 in this case. Table 2 shows the observed data, the expected cases under the logistic and Weibull models, and the values of the Hosmer-Lemeshow statistic. The X^2 test provides no evidence to reject the fit under either model.

TABLE II
Comparison of observed data and model predictions

	Subjects with abnormal neurological index		
Group[a]	Observed	Expected (Logistic)	Expected (Weibull)
1	0	0.79	0.071
2	0	0.69	0.069
3	0	0.70	0.12
4	0	0.73	0.34
5	2	0.92	0.88
6	1	1.1	1.8
7	3	1.4	2.5
8	4	3.3	4.2
9	5	5.2	5.2
10	7	7.2	6.7
Hosmer-Lemeshow goodness-of-fit X^2		7.2	3.0
p value		0.51	0.93

[a] Collapsed on percentiles of estimated probabilities.

Table III summarizes the excess risks associated with various maternal hair concentrations under different dose-response models. The table shows the results for the current dose-response analysis of the quantal data on neurologic effect index and similar analyses by Cox *et al.* (1989) of CNS signs and psychomotor retardation. The influence of the model choice can be observed by comparing the results for the logistic versus Weibull analyses of the neurologic index. At a maternal hair concentration of 1 ppm, the risk estimates under the two models differ by an order of magnitude. Changing the measure of health impact also affects the risk estimates. Risk estimates associated with the neurologic index differ by as much as a factor of 5 from those associated with CNS signs or psychomotor retardation, the endpoints selected by Cox *et al.* (1989).

TABLE III
Comparison of dose-response analyses

	Excess risk (%)					
	Present analysis Neurologic index		Cox *et al.* (1989) CNS signs		Cox *et al.*(1989) Psychomotor retardation	
Maternal hair Hg (ppm)	Logistic	Weibull	Logistic	Kernel smoothing	Logistic	Kernel smoothing
1	0.08	0.9	0.61	<0.5	0.52	<0.5
5	0.4	3.4	2.3	1	2.5	2
50	4.7	22	13	10	19	20

3. Assessment of Methylmercury Dose

Exposure to methylmercury for populations fishing in the Nechako Reservoir, Ogston Lake or Tezzeron Lake depends on the amount of fish consumed, the level of methylmercury contamination, and the body weight of the mother. Equation 3 shows the formula used to calculate maternal dose.

$$D_{MeHg} = \frac{C_{MeHg} \times I_F}{W_M} \tag{3}$$

where C_{MeHg} is the concentration of methylmercury in the fish (μg/g), I_F is the intake rate of fish (g/day), and W_M is the weight of the mother in kg. Miettenen (1973) found that 100% of ingested methylmercury is absorbed, so no parameter for absorption was included.

The concentration of methylmercury in trout is dependent on the size of trout, as the chemical accumulates in fish tissue over time. The linear relationships between size and mercury concentration were measured for trout from the Nechako Reservoir and Ogston and Tezzeron Lakes and found to be statistically significant. Bloom (1992) found that nearly 100% of the mercury in fish is in the methylated form. We therefore assumed that mercury concentration was equivalent to methylmercury concentration. The equations for the lines relating methylmercury concentration (C_{MeHg}) to fish weight (W_F) are given below.

Nechako Reservoir: $$C_{MeHg} = 0.078 + 0.11 \times W_F \quad (4)$$

Ogston Lake: $$C_{MeHg} = 0.12 + 0.020 \times W_F \quad (5)$$

Tezzeron Lake: $$C_{MeHg} = 0.049 + 0.13 \times W_F \quad (6)$$

Substituting fish weights in kilograms into equations (4), (5), and (6) will give the corresponding methylmercury concentrations in ppm. Uncertainty in the parameters of the lines could not be calculated directly from the data, because multiple measurements for a given size of fish were not generally made. To estimate uncertainty we used a nonparametric bootstrap data analysis technique (Efron and Gong, 1983; Efron and Tibshirani, 1993). For a given set of data, the residuals calculated in fitting the linear relationship were randomly added to the observed data and the slope and intercept recalculated. The process was used to produce 2,000 pairs of slopes and intercepts for each of the three bodies of water. In the Monte Carlo simulation of exposure, values for the slope and intercept were randomly selected from the 2,000 pairs of parameters.

To determine the concentration of methylmercury using the linear relationships above, we had to define the size of fish consumed. No information was available on the typical size of fish caught by anglers at the Nechako Reservoir or other lakes in the region. Triton (1991) collected data on the weights of fish from the reservoir, but these data cannot be interpreted to represent the true distribution of sizes. Although gillnets of various mesh sizes were used, any gear will have some size selectivity because of physical as well as behavioral differences between large and small fish (Hilborn and Walters, 1992). Further, these data do not indicate the typical sizes consumed, because anglers will tend to target the larger fish. To reflect these various uncertainties, we constructed a uniform distribution with the mean size ranging between 0.5 and 2.5 kg. The choice of a uniform distribution over this range is consistent with the data from the Nechako and with a study of an Ojibwa community in Ontario which found that the mean size of fish consumed was 1.3 kg (Hopper and Power, 1991).

Fish intake is another key parameter. Richardson and Currie (1993) conducted a large survey (n=2,538) of native women in Ontario who consumed fish from lakes over various seasons. The geometric mean fish consumption was 14.4 g/day, corresponding to an arithmetic mean of 27.2 g/day. The authors noted that this value for native fish consumption is lower than some other literature reports, but point out that many of the other surveys were based on limited samples taken over short periods of time. The mean value of freshwater fish intake observed in the Richardson and Currie study is 10-20 times the rate of freshwater fish consumption for the average Canadian, consistent with previous observations that natives consume greater quantities of fish. We selected

Richardson's and Currie's study as most relevant to our risk assessment, because of its careful design and size and the fact that the fish consumed were freshwater. We recognized that only a portion of the fish consumed would be contaminated with methylmercury to any significant level, so we had to adjust the fish consumption values to reflect this. Quantitative information on the relative amounts of various species consumed by natives from the reservoir and lakes in the region were not available. A Health and Welfare Canada (1993) study indicated that the favorite fish of the local band was salmon, which is relatively uncontaminated by methylmercury. The Columbia River Inter-Tribal Fish Commission (CRIFC, 1994) reported that 26% percent of the total fish consumed by native anglers were resident fish, which are most likely to contain locally important contaminants. Because this information may be specific to the region and tribal customs, we chose to make a conservative assumption that 50% of the fish consumed by the target population is contaminated.

Table IV summarizes the values of the variable and fixed parameters assumed in the dose calculation. We constructed estimated distributions of methylmercury exposure by generating 10,000 estimates of dose for each of the three bodies of water using Monte Carlo simulation.

TABLE IV
Summary of parameters used in probabilistic risk assessment

A. Distributions

Parameter	Mean	Standard deviation or range	Shape of distribution	Comments
Female body weight	62.0 kg	11.1 kg	Normal	Canadian Environmental Health Directorate (1993)
Fish consumption	14.4 g/day (geometric) (arithmetic mean = 27.2 g/day)	3.1 g/day (geometric)	Lognormal	From Richardson and Currie (1993) study of 2,538 women from reserves in Ontario consuming freshwater fish.
Size of fish consumed	1.5 kg	0.5-2.5	Uniform	Consistent with tail end of data distribution from Nechako Reservoir and study of an Ojibwa community (Hopper and Power, 1991).

TABLE IV (continued)

B. Fixed parameters

Parameter	Value	Comments
Fraction of mercury in fish present as methylmercury	1	Bloom *et al.* (1992)
Fraction of ingested methylmercury absorbed	1	Miettinen (1973)
Correlation between body weight and fish consumption	0.33	From a Canadian survey cited by Lipfert *et al.* (1996).
Fraction of fish consumed that contain mercury	0.5	Salmon (unaffected by local mercury contamination) is favorite species of natives in region (HWC, 1993). An assumption that half the fish consumed are contaminated is conservative, based on data from Columbia River Basin (CRIFC, 1994).

The study of Iraqi mothers and children (Marsh *et al.*, 1987) that we used in the dose-response analysis measured peak maternal hair mercury during pregnancy as a biomarker for methylmercury exposure. In order to characterize risks , we converted methylmercury dose predicted for mothers consuming fish from the Nechako Reservoir, Ogston Lake or Tezzeron Lake to peak hair concentration using a series of factors determined empirically by Kershaw *et al.* (1980) and Kjellstrom *et al.* (1989).

$$B_{Hg} = \frac{D_{MeHg} \times (62.4 \pm 3.7)}{1000} \qquad (7)$$

$$H_{Hg\text{-}mean} = B_{Hg} \times (292 \pm 84) \qquad (8)$$

$$H_{Hg\text{-}peak} = H_{Hg\text{-}mean} \times (1.5 \pm 0.37) \qquad (9)$$

where B_{Hg} is the mean blood level of mercury in µg/ml, D_{MeHg} is the ingested dose of methylmercury in µg/kg-day, $H_{Hg\text{-}mean}$ and $H_{Hg\text{-}peak}$ are the mean and peak levels of mercury in the hair in µg/g (ppm). We combined the estimated dose-response relationships with the predicted peak maternal hair concentrations in a Monte Carlo simulation to generate risk distributions.

4. Results

Table V summarizes the mean dose and hair levels derived from the estimated exposure distributions for natives consuming fish from the reservoir and two lakes. The predicted dose and hair levels are identical for the Nechako Reservoir and Tezzeron Lake. As expected, exposure to methylmercury is somewhat lower for natives consuming fish from Ogston Lake. None of the exposures differ significantly from those estimated by the World Health Organization (WHO, 1990) or Fleming *et al.* (1995) for the general population.

We compared our predicted exposure values to measured hair levels for natives living in the region. A survey of mercury hair levels in the Cheslatta band was conducted by Health and Welfare Canada (1993). The Cheslatta live south of Francois Lake and fish in waters impacted by the Nechako Reservoir. The 26 individuals studied were found to have hair levels within Health and Welfare Canada's acceptable limit of 6 ppm, with the highest measured value at 2.1 ppm. We calculated the mean hair level by substituting one half the detection limit for the 14 samples below the detection limit (0.5 ppm). We converted the hair levels to estimated dose following equations (7) and (8). Results of these calculations are summarized in Table V. Our predicted hair levels and mean doses are consistent with those for the Cheslatta, suggesting that the assumptions selected for exposure parameters in our model were reasonable.

TABLE V
Mean methylmercury exposure levels

	Mean dose (μg/kg-day)	Mean hair Hg (μg/g)
Nechako Reservoir	0.05	0.9
Tezzeron Lake	0.05	0.9
Ogston Lake	0.03	0.5
General population		
WHO (1990)	0.04	0.7
Fleming *et al.* (1995), Ontario	0.02	0.4
Cheslatta band (n=26)	~0.03	~0.5

We measured risk as the probability of an abnormal neurological index ($P^{(1)}$). Table VI summarizes mean and upper bound risks associated with the reservoir and two lakes and estimated mean risks for the general population. The distributions of risks are identical for the Nechako Reservoir and Tezzeron Lake, as expected from the exposure analysis. Due to the somewhat elevated concentrations of mercury in the fish from these two bodies of water, the predicted risks are slightly higher than those for Ogston Lake. The mean risks predicted for all three bodies of water are comparable to those for the general population, suggesting that this target population is not experiencing significant risk for neurologic dysfunction.

TABLE VI
Excess mean and upper bound risks

	Excess risk[a]			
	Logistic		Weibull	
	Mean	Upper 95%	Mean	Upper 95%
Nechako	0.001	0.004	0.01	0.03
Tezzeron Lake	0.001	0.004	0.01	0.03
Ogston Lake	0.0007	0.002	0.007	0.02
General population				
WHO (1990)	0.0009		0.009	
Fleming *et al.* (1995) Ontario	0.0005		0.005	

[a] The logistic model predicts a risk of 0.0976 at zero dose; excess risks due to mercury intake were calculated by subtracting this background. The Weibull model predicts zero risk at zero dose, so no adjustment was necessary.

5. Conclusions

We have described the correlated measurements of methylmercury's effect on neurological development with a single index. Normal and abnormal levels of the index were defined and related to the mercury concentration in maternal hair. Both the logistic and Weibull models were consistent with the dose-response data. Risks of neurologic effect predicted for various maternal hair concentrations vary significantly depending on the choice of dose-response model and how the health impact is measured. Recent results from studies of chronic fish consumers in the Seychelles (Cox *et al.*, 1996) and Faroe Islands (Weihe *et al.*, 1996) may provide better information on the risks of low-dose methylmercury exposures.

We find that potential health risks to native populations consuming fish from the Nechako Reservoir are comparable to those associated with other lakes in the region, as well as to mean risks for the general population. Native populations consuming typical quantities of fish from these bodies of water are not likely to experience elevated risks for neurologic disorder in their children.

Acknowledgements

We thank Brian Wheatley and Ron Wyzga for encouraging us to submit this paper. Special thanks to Kevin McCreight, Dave Warburton and Christina Economos for preparing Figure 1. This research was supported in part by Alcan Smelters & Chemicals Ltd.

References

Bloom, N.S.: 1992, *Can. J. Fish. Aquat. Sci.* **49**, 1010-1017.

Canadian Environmental Health Directorate: 1993, *Reference Values for Canadian Populations*, prepared by the Environmental Health Directorate Working Group on Reference Values.

Columbia River Inter-Tribal Fish Commission (CRIFC): 1994, *A Fish Consumption Survey of the Umatilla, Nez Perce, Yakama, and Warm Springs Tribes of the Columbia River Basin*, report no. 94-3, Portland, Oregon.

Cox, C., Myers, G., Davidson, P.W., Cernichiari, E., Choi, A., Ping, G., Axtell, C.D., Shamlaye, C., Marsh, D.O., Berlin, M., and Clarkson, T.W.: 1996, *The Seychelles Child Development Study: Longitudinal Analysis of Developmental Outcomes from Testing at Six Months, Nineteen Months, and Twenty-Nine Months*, presented at Fourth International Conference on Mercury as a Global Pollutant, Hamburg, Germany.

Cox, C., Clarkson, T.W., Marsh, D.O., Amin-Zaki, L., Tikriti, S. and Myers, G.: 1989, *Environ. Res.* **49**, 318-322.

Efron, B. and Gong, G.: 1983, *Amer. Stat.* **37**, 36-48.

Efron, B. and Tibshirani, R.J.: 1993, *An Introduction to the Bootstrap*, Chapman and Hall, New York.

Fleming, S.W., Radzius, L.V., and Ursitti, F.: 1995, *Health Risk Assessment of Mercury Contamination in the Vicinity of ICI Forest Products, Cornwall, Ontario*, report no. 95-06312, prepared for Ontario Ministry of Environment and Energy.

Health and Welfare Canada (HWC): 1993, *Mercury Survey - 1992: Cheslatta Indian Band and Area Residents*, Occupational and Environmental Health Program, Medical Services Branch, Health and Welfare Canada.

Hilborn, R. and Walters, C.J.: 1992, *Quantitative Fisheries Stock Assessment: Choice, Dynamics and Uncertainty*, Chapman and Hall, New York.

Hopper, M. and Power, G.: 1991., *Arctic* **44**(4), 267-274.

Hosmer, D.W. and Lemeshow, S.: 1989, *Applied Logistic Regression*, Wiley-Interscience, New York.

Jackson, T.A.: 1988, *Can. J. Fish. Aquat. Sci.* **45**, 97-121.

Kershaw, T.G., Dhahir, P.H., and Clarkson, T.W.: 1980, *Arch. Environ. Health* **35**(1), 28-36.

Kjellstrom, T., Kennedy, P., Wallis, S., Stewart, A., Friberg, L., Lind, B., Wutherspoon, T., and Mantell, C.: 1989, *Physical and Mental Development of Children with Prenatal Exposure to Mercury from Fish, Stage 2: Interviews and Psychological Tests at Age 6*, Report 3642, National Swedish Environmental Protection Board, Solna, Sweden.

Lipfert, F.W., Moskowitz, P.D., Fthenakis, V., and Saroff, L.: 1996, *Neurotox.* **17**(1), 197-212.

Marsh, D.O., Clarkson, T.W., Cox, C., Myers, G.J., Amin-Zaki, L. and Al-Tikriti, S: 1987, *Arch. Neurol.*, **44**, 1017-1022.

Miettinen, J.K.: 1973, *Absorption and elimination of dietary mercury (Hg^{2+}) and methyl mercury in man*. In: Miller, M.W. and Clarkson, T.W., ed., *Mercury, Mercurials and Mercaptans*, C.C. Thomas, Springfield, 233-240.

Morgan, M.G. and Henrion, M.: 1990, *Uncertainty. A Guide to Dealing with Uncertainty in Quantitative Risk and Policy Analysis*, Cambridge University Press, Cambridge.

Richardson, G.M. and Currie, D.J. :1993, *J. of Exp. Anal. and Environ. Epi.* **3**(1), 23-38.

Selvin, S: 1995, *Practical Biostatistical Methods*, Duxbury Press, London.

Stata Corporation: 1993, *Stata®: Statistics, Graphics and Data Management*. College Station, Texas.

Triton Environmental Consultants Ltd.: 1991, *Survey of Mercury Levels in Nechako Reservoir, British Columbia, 1991*, prepared for Alcan Smelters & Chemicals Ltd., Vancouver, B.C.

Triton Environmental Consultants Ltd: 1992, *Evaluation of Mercury Concentration in Selected Environmental Receptors in the Williston Lake and Peace River Areas of British Columbia*, prepared for Environmental Resources, B.C. Hydro, Vancouver, B.C.
Weihe, P., Grandjean, P., Debes, F., Sorensen, N., and White, R.F.: 1996, *Neurotoxic Potential of Prenatal Exposure to Methylmercury: A Cohort Study in the Faroe Islands*, presented at Fourth International Conference on Mercury as a Global Pollutant, Hamburg, German.
World Health Organization (WHO): 1990, *Environmental Health Criteria 101, Methylmercury*, WHO, Geneva.

ESTIMATING EXPOSURE TO METHYLMERCURY: EFFECTS OF UNCERTAINTIES

FREDERICK W. LIPFERT

1Department of Applied Science, Brookhaven National Laboratory, Upton, NY 11973.

(Received January 9, 1997; accepted January 13, 1997)

Abstract. Uncertainties in exposures can lead to biased estimates of slopes and thresholds in the exposure-response relationships that are developed from regression analysis. This paper reviews published exposure and epidemiological studies of methylmercury (MeHg) from the perspective of the accuracy and precision of the estimates used to represent the actual doses received. Sources of such uncertainties, collectively referred to as "exposure errors", include instrumental and analytical errors, sampling and survey uncertainties, and individual variability in the relationships between the exposure metrics and the actual doses to target organs. Because the relationship between maternal intake and the consequent dose to the fetal brain varies among individuals, epidemiological studies of the effects of prenatal exposure must necessarily be accompanied by larger exposure uncertainties than comparable studies of effects on the mothers. The increased exposure errors typically result in attenuated slopes of the dose-response functions and under-estimates of thresholds, so that part of the apparent increased sensitivity of the fetus that has been developed from epidemiological studies may in fact be due to their inherently less certain exposures. Sources and magnitudes of exposure error found in the literature are discussed and their statistical ramifications are explored with Monte Carlo simulations. The paper also finds that, after adjusting for exposure error, the relationship between dietary intake and blood concentration is consistent with an average half-life shorter than has typically been used and that using population averages yields a consistent but sub-linear relationship between dietary intake of Hg and hair concentration. Investigators are urged to obtain (and present) data on more than one exposure metric, so that their relative uncertainties may be assessed independently.

1. Introduction

Mercury is a neurotoxic pollutant that occurs in the environment in both inorganic and organic forms. Human health effects are manifested mainly through eating foods containing methylmercury (MeHg); ingestion of contaminated fish is now the most important exposure pathway. Rates of dietary intake are used for exposure control, by means of fish consumption advisories, for example. Several epidemiological studies have attempted to define the onset and severity of human responses to MeHg by using certain biomarkers as indices of exposure, in addition to the traditional measures of dietary intake. This paper explores the statistical ramifications of the uncertainties and biases inherent in these various exposure metrics for MeHg.

"Exposure error" is defined here as the difference between the surrogate measure used in an epidemiological study and the actual dose to the target organ, i.e., the brain. These "errors" (in a statistical sense) thus include measurement errors and also individual variabilities, which are not really errors *per se*. The paper begins by reviewing well-established metabolic relationships, as applied to transient and steady exposures. The statistical ramifications of uncertainties in exposures are outlined, and then some specific examples from extant studies are reviewed. Relationships between common exposure measures are discussed, as examples of the underlying uncertainties. A consistent but sublinear relationship is shown between hair Hg concentrations and MeHg intake rates based on averages obtained from various studies of fish eating populations.

1.1 MeHg METABOLISM

The relationships between intake rates of methylmercury and subsequent concentrations of biomarkers are defined by metabolic processes that have been studied more thoroughly than those of almost any other toxic air pollutant (WHO, 1990). MeHg is efficiently and nearly completely absorbed in the intestine and enters the bloodstream within a few hours, from which it is widely distributed throughout the body. Its presence in the body may be described by a first-order decay process, in which the rate of loss through excretion is proportional to the remaining concentration. The time-dependent concentration is defined by:

$$C = m(1-e^{-kt})/k \tag{1}$$

where C is the concentration, m is the daily intake rate, assumed to be steady, t is the elapsed time in days, k is the elimination constant given by $\ln(2)/t_{1/2}$, and $t_{1/2}$ is the half-life of MeHg in the body. At equilibrium, $C = m/k$. It is commonly assumed that concentrations in blood or the whole-body average concentration, referred to as "body burden," may be used as surrogates for the actual dose to the brain. Conversion from body-burden to blood concentration requires an estimate of the fraction of MeHg body burden taken up by blood, often assumed to be about 5-7%, and the ratio of blood volume to body mass (about 0.07 L/kg).

After ingestion stops, C decreases according to:

$$C/C_{max} = e^{-kt} \tag{2}$$

Detailed experiments using radiolabeled MeHg in fish ingested by 15 volunteers (Miettinen, 1972) showed an initial high rate of excretion for a few days before the steady model described by (1) and (2) pertains. Decay rates have been measured to estimate $t_{1/2}$, which varies substantially among individuals. Many studies show that Hg concentrations in scalp hair track those in blood quite closely with a lag of about a few weeks, providing a temporal record of exposure over the length of hair available for analysis.

1.2 STEADY-STATE VS. TRANSIENT EXPOSURES

The primary concerns about MeHg exposure involve steady, long-term consumption of contaminated fish in which excretion of MeHg equals intake and tissue concentrations are constant over time (i.e., in equilibrium). However, transient poisoning incidents in the past have provided much of the information that has been used in assessing such risks. One of the richest sources of epidemiological information on the health effects of MeHg is the grain poisoning episode of 1971-72 in Iraq (Bakir *et al.*, 1973), in which rural villagers ate bread made from seed grain treated with MeHg fungicides. Consumption occurred over a few weeks to a few months, and there were many deaths and hospitalizations; had consumption continued longer, the overall effects of the incident undoubtedly would have been far worse. Since individual ingestion rates differed in terms of duration as well as intensity, this data set may be more heterogeneous than those obtained from studies of fish-eating populations. Because blood samples were obtained up to 131 days after ingestion stopped, the data must be adjusted to account for losses due to excretion (Eq. 2). Such corrections are uncertain because of the extremely variable half-lives in this population (as measured in hair by Al-Shahristani and Shihab, 1974). In addition, in that study, length of ingestion was positively correlated with blood concentration. Unfortunately, Bakir et al. reported dose-response data only in terms of group averages of about 20 individuals; the inherent within-group variability would lead to further uncertainties in these relationships. Even the "unexposed" persons that comprise the lower end of the Iraqi dose-response curves may have had some exposure, as shown by the variability in their hair Hg concentration profiles.

Englender *et al.* (1980) discussed an extended family who ate eggs over a period up to 50-55 days from hens that were fed on Hg-contaminated grain. There was an excellent relationship (R=0.92) between family members' blood Hg (determined by atomic absorption) and their estimated daily rate of egg consumption, but the blood concentrations were much lower than might have been expected from the Iraqi incident. For example, the maximum MeHg individual intake rate was about 20 ug/kg/d, which would correspond to a total intake of about 70 mg of MeHg. However, in this individual, the blood concentration was only 20 ug/L four days after consumption stopped and the Iraqi experience (Figure 5 in Bakir *et al.*, 1973) would have predicted a blood concentration of over 500 ug/L. Thus, it appears that transient responses may differ markedly among individuals.

One major disadvantage of short-term (non-equilibrium) exposures is their relative insensitivity to the half-life of the agent in question. As seen from Eq. 1. a longer half-life results in a higher equilibrium concentration of MeHg, for a given steady level of intake. Figure 1 (based on Eq. 1) compares the ratio of body burden to intake rate over a range of half-lives and ingestion periods typical of the Iraqi incident. It shows that steady-state populations will reflect uncertainties in half-life much more than short-term experiments such as the Iraqi incident. Also indicated on Figure 1 are the half-life (76 days) that has been used in many analyses, including the risk analysis of Lipfert *et al.* (1994, 1996), and a more recent revised value of 44 days (Smith *et al.*, 1994). Smith and Farris (1996) recently proposed a more complicated pharmacokinetic model that results in MeHg half-lives of 51-56 days. These 30-40% uncertainties in half-life translate into proportional uncertainties in the severity of neurological effects for a given MeHg intake rate.

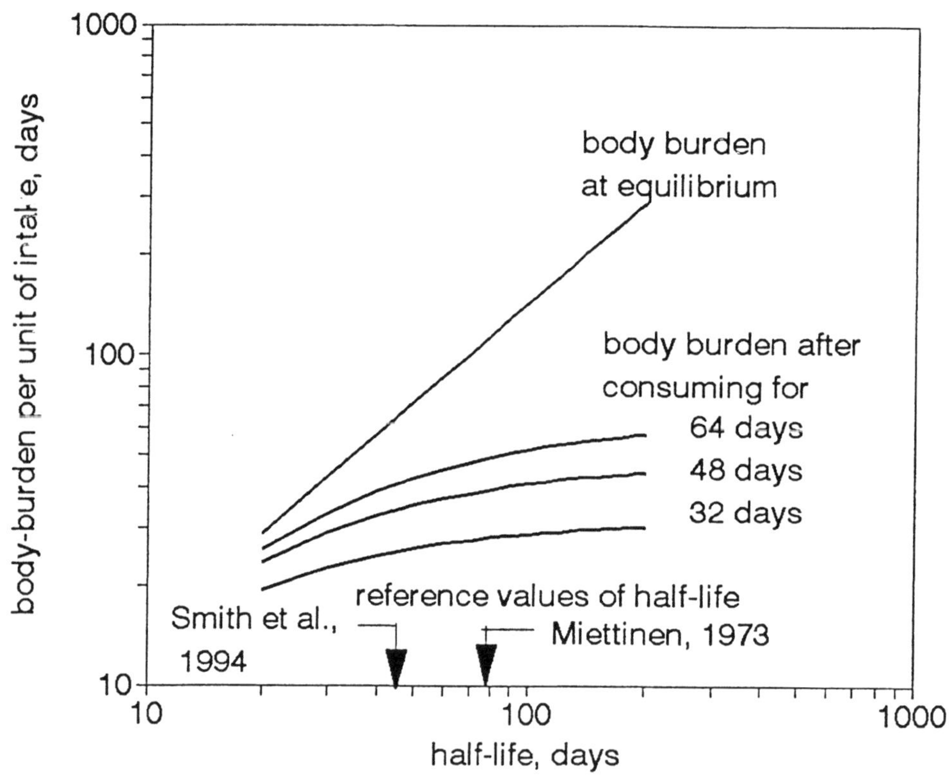

Fig. 1. Simulation of the effects of various assumed half-lives of MeHg on retention in the body, for selected lengths of exposure time and at equilibrium. Typical reference values of MeHg half life are also shown.

1.3 IMPLICATIONS OF UNCERTAIN EXPOSURE ESTIMATES

The statistical consequences of an imperfect measure of exposure in an epidemiological study include reduced measures of regression "fit" and biased estimates of slope (Sherlock and Quinn, 1988). When exposure errors are normally distributed, the bias in the slope (towards the null) is given by the square of the coefficient of correlation between the true and surrogate exposure measures. For a linear regression model, underestimating the slope also biases the threshold towards the left (Figure 2); for shallow slopes, i.e. weak effects, the underestimate of the threshold becomes substantial, In this simulated case, the underestimate of the threshold is about 65% of the mean exposure. In multivariate regressions, in which the effects of Hg intake are contrasted with those of potential confounders, it is just as important to represent the confounding factors accurately as it is to measure the MeHg exposure accurately (Thomas *et al.*, 1993). In addition, errors in exposure measurement can obscure the true shape of the dose-response function (Thomas *et al.*, 1993).

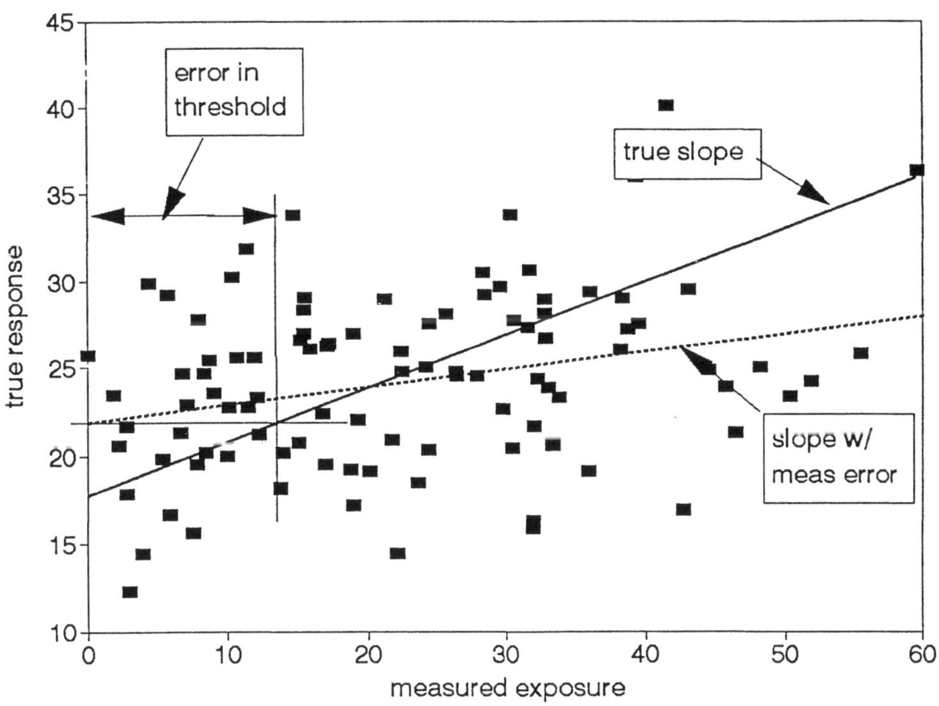

Fig. 2. Illustrations of some typical effects of exposure uncertainty on dose-response functions. In this example, 100 observations are shown with the true (underlying) dose-response relationship, and with the relationship that would be obtained if the correlation between the surrogate and true exposures were 0.55.

Because fetal exposures cannot be measured directly during gestation and the individual mother-infant MeHg relationships vary, epidemiological studies of the effects of prenatal exposures on infant and childhood development must inevitably work with imperfect surrogates for the actual dose to the fetal brain. The physiological characteristics of both mother and child are involved, and thus the distribution of fetal exposure errors will be wider than those corresponding to exposures of the mothers. In addition, the most critical timing of fetal MeHg exposure is not well established, and determining this timing from maternal hair requires knowledge of the concentration lag with respect to fetal exposure and the rate of growth of maternal hair. For example, Cernichiari *et al.* (1995a) showed correlations around 0.6-0.8 between Hg concentrations in maternal hair (reflecting conditions at delivery) and in 27 autopsied infant brains; this would result in a downward bias in the slope of a maternal hair-based exposure-response function of about 50%. Grandjean et al. (1992) show similar scatter in the relationships between cord blood Hg and maternal hair Hg, for a much larger cohort (about 1000). Such uncertainties result either in a threshold that is too low, in the case of a hockey-stick function, or a logistic response curve that is too shallow (overpredicting the low risks and underpredicting the high ones). An example of the latter effect is shown in Figure 3, in which the relationship found by Myers et al. in the Seychelles Islands pilot study has been adjusted upward to account for the (typical) 0.7 correlation between MeHg levels in maternal hair and in infant brains. This adjustment has only minor effects at low doses, but it makes the upper end of the curve (which has been extrapolated well beyond Myers et al.'s data) more closely resemble the Iraqi data.

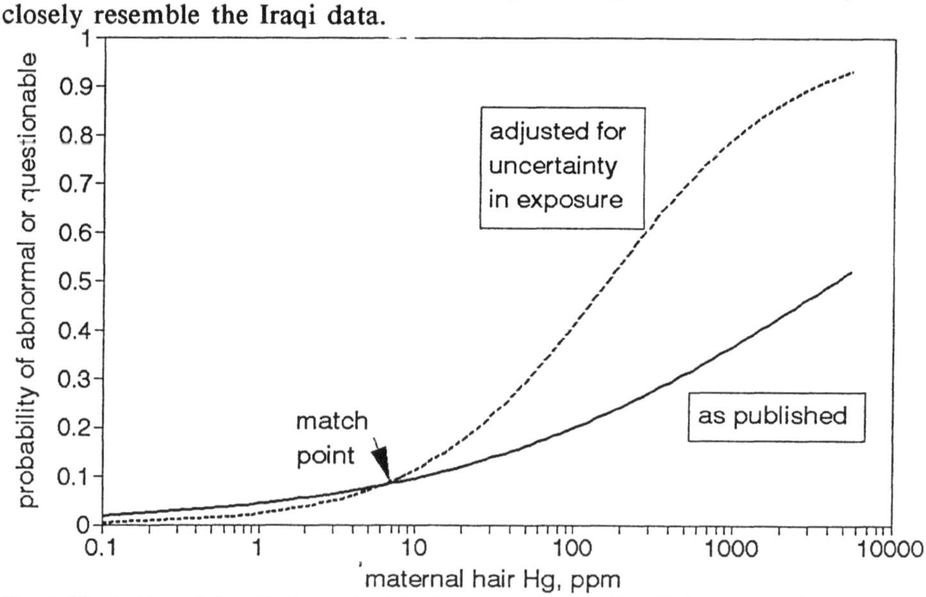

Fig. 3. Illustration of the effect on a logistic dose-response function (taken from Myers et al., 1995) of correction for a 50% bias due to uncertainties in actual exposures.

Thus, studies of the effects of prenatal exposures should be expected to yield dose-response functions that are inherently more biased than those from comparable studies of adults, *ceteris paribus*. This greater bias will shift the apparent threshold for the onset of congenital effects to the left, providing the appearance of a lower margin of safety with respect to MeHg intake levels.

2. MeHg Exposure Metrics and Their Statistical Problems

Each of these three measures of exposure (dietary intake rate, blood concentration, and hair concentration) offers certain advantages and disadvantages for an epidemiological study. According to Spitzer *et al.* (1988), "No perfect measure of exposure is available," which is interpreted to mean that none actually represents the dose to the adult or fetal brain. Intake of MeHg is a direct measure and represents the means of controlling exposure; however, intake rates are difficult to ascertain accurately for each member of a large population because of variations in MeHg concentrations in fish and uncertain recall of past consumption. Studies of children may find it necessary to distinguish between fetal exposures, for which no direct measures are available, and postnatal ingestion exposures.

Blood MeHg may be measured accurately but requires an invasive procedure and gives only a snapshot of the MeHg concentration at the time of sampling; blood concentrations may be temporarily elevated just after eating fish, for example, and thus umbilical cord blood may not reflect the fetal brain dose at the most critical time during gestation. Thus, blood data are most useful when dietary intake rates are known to be steady (which may be difficult to determine). Hair Hg concentrations can provide an integrated record of MeHg along the length of the hair, but the constants of proportionality with blood Hg, body burden, or intake vary among individuals; also, there may be within-person variability (Al-Shahristani and Al-Haddad, 1973). Hair concentrations and dietary intake thus appear to be the main candidates for estimating long-term fluctuating exposures.

2.1 MEASUREMENT RELIABILITY OF Hg HAIR CONCENTRATIONS

Sources of uncertainty in inferring exposures from measured hair concentrations for individuals include the instrumental and analysis methods used, contamination by external agents such as hair preparations, heterogeneity on the scalp, and uncertainties in rates of hair growth and thus the timing of exposure. Specific problems may arise from the quantities of hair required for reliable analysis, smearing of peaks in individual strands, and averaging over time. In addition, hair/blood Hg concentration ratios and hair concentration/intake ratios vary among individuals. The lag in maternal hair concentrations with respect to blood concentrations must be accounted for in estimating fetal exposures. However, Marsh *et al.* (1995) reported correlations of 0.90-0.95 between maternal and infant hair Hg in a fish-consuming population.

Methods of analysis for Hg in hair have improved since the early methods used by the Japanese investigating Minamata disease. The dithizon (colorimetric) method used during the 1960s is thought to be unreliable at low concentrations (WHO, 1990). Neutron activation analysis used in early hair analyses in Iraq (Al-Shahristani and Al-Haddad, 1973) may also have had some reliability problems at that time (J.C. Smith, personal communication, August 1996). Marsh *et al.* (1987) used X-ray fluorescence (calibrated against atomic absorption analysis) with single strands of hair from Iraqi mothers to better estimate peak MeHg levels during pregnancy; however, such peaks may not always occur at the most critical times for fetal development.

Al-Shahristani and Al-Haddad (1973) reported replicate measurements of hair Hg from an Iraqi individual not thought to have eaten contaminated grain. Longitudinal Hg profiles were shown from three different areas of the head. While the three were qualitatively similar, one profile had Hg levels about a factor of three higher than the others. The median concentrations and geometric standard deviations (GSDs) in the three scalp areas were (6.15, 1.39), (5.23, 1.71), and (17.8, 2.36); the three rates of hair growth also appeared differ slightly. The precision of the method (neutron activation) appeared to be excellent in terms of repeated measurements on the same sample; the minimum hair concentration in the "high" area was about same as the minimum in the other two areas. The degree of variability in this individual is similar to that found in a population. Also, the average values of about 6 ug/g (and even the minimum levels of about 4 ug/g) seem high for an "unexposed" individual, but the shapes of the spikes in the longitudinal profiles do not suggest prolonged MeHg ingestion. Thus a high bias is suspected in at least some of the Iraqi hair Hg data due to randomly high measurements.

Experiments showing that the MeHg sequestered in hair appears to be stable and impervious to washing (Al-Shahristani and Al-Haddad, 1973) provide some confidence on the underlying precision of measurement. Usually, the overwhelming portion of total Hg in hair is organic (MeHg), so that total Hg often is used as a more convenient exposure metric. There appear to be only small differences according to hair color (Eads and Lambdin, 1973), but males tend to have slightly higher hair Hg levels (Shimomura *et al.*, 1980), perhaps because of higher dietary intake (Al-Shahristani *et al.*, 1976). Sky-Peck and Joseph (1983) found that a group of 24 black females had about half the Hg hair content of Caucasians and Asians, but this could have been due to dietary differences.

Some epidemiological studies have used peak rather than average hair Hg concentrations during pregnancy (Marsh *et al.*, 1987). For example, Kjellstrom *et al.* (1986, 1989) recommended using a ratio of 1.5 to convert from mean to peak hair Hg concentrations. However, Marsh *et al.* (1995) found close correspondence between peak and mean measures in mothers in a Peruvian fishing village (means of 8.34 vs. 7.05 ug/g, for a ratio of 1.18). The correlation between the two measures was not given but appeared to be quite high based on the other statistics given. It thus appears that variability in peak/mean ratios of hair Hg concentration (as well as the most critical timing of peaks during pregnancy) creates further sources of exposure uncertainty.

2.2 RELIABILITY OF DIETARY ESTIMATES

Estimates of dietary intake of MeHg can be problematic. The preferred metric is the daily intake per unit of body mass (ug/kg/d), which can be estimated from the Hg content of fish, the average meal size, the frequency of consumption, and the body mass. Hg content and consumption frequency are probably the most variable of these parameters. In this paper, 70 kg is assumed for the average body mass for adult North Americans and Europeans, 50 kg for the Iraqis studied by Bakir *et al.* (1973), and 60 kg for other populations, unless otherwise specified.

Lipfert *et al.* (1994, 1996) recognized that the variability of the Hg content of individual fish meals is not an issue for long-term health effects, since each meal represents only an incremental contribution to the equilibrium body burden. Thus, body burdens for the more frequent fish eaters will tend to more nearly reflect the overall average fish Hg content and meal size for the population than for infrequent consumers. This phenomenon was modeled by an empirical equation that decreased the variability of intake as the frequency of consumption increased.

An additional source of variability is the rate of consumption. Fish meals comprise a Poisson distribution (variance=mean), for which relative variability is most important at low consumption rates. Figure 4 illustrates this relative variability of dietary intake as a function of consumption frequency, based on the following assumptions (CI = confidence interval; GSD = geometric standard deviation).

1. Fish meals average 200 g with a standard deviation of 40 g.
2. The median (individual) fish Hg content is 0.15 ug/g with 95% CIs of 0.019 and 1.21 ug/g (GSD = 3.0). GSD decreases with increasing meal frequency.
3. The mean body mass is 73 kg with 95% CIs of 47 and 113 kg (GSD = 1.26).

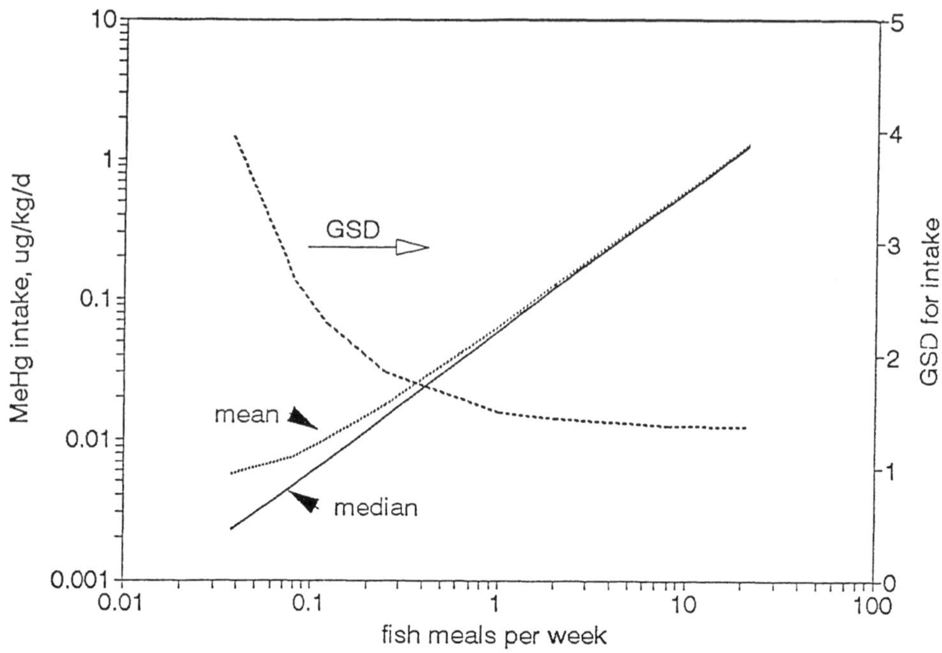

Fig. 4. Illustrative plot of variability in dietary intake of MeHg, Monte Carlo simulations at each of several assumed rates of fish consumption. The variability among individuals in the simulated group of 1000 is indicated by the geometric standard deviation (GSD) scale on the right. Simulations assume a Poisson distribution of fish meal events and the following mean values: fish meal mass, 200 g; body mass, 71 kg; Hg, 0.15 ug/g.

In order to illustrate the ramifications of this degree of variability, Monte Carlo simulations of 1000 trials each were run over a range of mean fish meal frequencies, from twice a year to three times daily; the results were plotted in Figure 4. The figure shows that intake variability (as expressed by its GSD, right-hand axis) is minimal for consumption frequencies exceeding about one meal every two weeks, implying that the variability in fish Hg content becomes the dominant factor in the variability of dietary intake. Also, under these assumptions, it is unlikely for the mean dietary intake rate of MeHg to exceed about 1 ug/kg/d. The estimated mean intakes would scale linearly with median fish Hg concentration; for example, a population consuming from a fish population with a median Hg concentration of 0.75 ug/g would be unlikely to exceed a mean intake rate of about 5 ug/kg/d.

For children, breast milk also constitutes a source of (postnatal) MeHg exposure (Grandjean *et al.*, 1995), in addition to fish consumption. Thus, it may be difficult to distinguish whether any childhood neurological defects are due to prenatal rather than childhood exposures (or to some combination), depending on the relative reliability of each of these exposure estimates.

3. Interrelationships Among MeHg Exposure Measures

One way of evaluating the reliability of estimates of MeHg exposure is to examine how well various measures relate to one another within a given study, using regression analysis. Random noise in the dependent variable will give a poorer fit, but the relationship will remain unbiased. However, random noise in the independent variable will also bias the slope towards the null, as discussed above. It should be axiomatic that knowledge of the reliability of the exposure measurements is required to properly interpret any epidemiological study.

As indicated above, there is a well-established protocol for estimating the body burden and blood concentration that would result from a specified rate of dietary intake of MeHg. However, predictions of the ensuing hair concentrations are based purely on empirical data. Since hair concentration has become the exposure metric of choice for studies of congenital effects, the reliability of the hair/blood or hair/intake relationship becomes important.

In previous simulations (Lipfert *et al.*, 1996, hereafter referred to as the "BNL model") derived the following ratios among median (geometric mean) exposure estimates for the two scenarios that were analyzed:

blood/intake:	69, 74	(ug/L per ug/kg/d)
hair/intake:	17.6, 18.3	(ug/g per ug/kg/d)
hair/blood:	0.255, 0.247	(ug/g per ug/L)

In the following sections, the various experimental determinations are compared with these "benchmark" values.

3.1 BLOOD AND HAIR MERCURY CONCENTRATIONS VS. INTAKE

Birke *et al.* (1972) developed relationships among intake, blood, and hair Hg concentrations in a small group of Swedish subjects by estimating their fish consumption rates and the typical Hg content of the species consumed. Given the relatively crude estimates of intake, their relationship with blood Hg is almost suspiciously good:

blood Hg (ug/L) = 56 intake (ug/kg/d)
(n=6, R=0.995, forced through the origin).

The relationship with hair fit only slightly less well:

hair Hg (ug/g) = 14.4 intake (ug/kg/d)
(n=7, R=0.91, forced through the origin).

However, log-log scatter plots suggested a linear relationship between blood Hg and intake, but the corresponding relationship for hair Hg was closer to a 3/4 power law. The hair/blood regression slope was 0.286; individual hair/blood ratios ranged from 0.14 to 0.59.

Skerfving (1974) followed this study with a slightly larger one, based on blood cell Hg concentrations, rather than whole blood. Using the tabulated data of Birke *et al.* for both parameters, the conversion factor is

concentration in whole blood = 0.54 (concentration in blood cells). (3)

Converting Skerfving's regression to a whole blood basis yields

(whole) blood Hg (ug/L) = 11 + 38 intake (ug/kg/d) (n=22, R=0.96)

The slope factor of 38 is lower than expected but the high correlation coefficient does not suggest errors in dietary measurements; the intercept suggests a relatively high concentration of inorganic mercury in blood. The data points were read from Skerfving's Figure 4 and some alternative regressions were computed. First, forcing the regression through the origin raises the slope factor to 41; the inverse regression yielded a slope factor of 44 (ug/L)/(ug/kg/d). Using a log-log model yielded the relationship

(whole) blood Hg (ug/L) = 58 intake$^{0.785}$ (R=0.98) (4)

The exponent 0.785 had a standard error of 0.04 and thus was significantly different from unity, but this finding may depend on the low values that were difficult to read precisely from the published graph.

Two separate regressions (by age group) of blood Hg on estimated total intake (dose) were used by Bakir *et al.* (1973) in estimating the body burdens used in their dose-response functions. A better procedure would be to pool the age-specific data and use dose per unit of body weight. Since blood measurements are likely to be more precise than the dose estimates, it might be preferable to perform the inverse regression instead. Using an average period of ingestion of 48.6 days, the direct regression produced a slope of 21 ug/L per ug/kg/d, while the inverse regression yielded 33 ug/L per ug/kg/d (after "re-inversion"). Using an ingestion period of 60 days to correspond to the higher exposures would increase the inverse slope to about 41, in conformance with other studies. These "corrections" are in the opposite direction from that implied by the methodology of Miettinen (1972) that was discussed by Bakir *et al.*

Sherlock *et al.* (1982) developed the following relationship between total blood Hg and dietary intake:

$$\text{blood Hg (ug/L)} = 5.68 + 0.18 \text{ dietary intake (ug/d)} \qquad (R=0.54)$$

After adjusting the intake variable to ug/kg/d (70 kg mean), if it is assumed that all of the error is in the dietary variable as suggested by Sherlock and Quinn (1988) and divide the slope by R^2, the adjusted relationship would be:

$$\text{blood Hg (ug/L)} = 1.9 + 43 \text{ dietary intake (ug/d)} \qquad (5)$$

which is considerably closer to expectations. Using this procedure on Haxton *et al.*'s data (1979) yields adjusted slopes of 42 and 48 for the two English communities they studied. Thus, the combined range of the linear proportionality constants relating steady dietary intake to equilibrium blood concentration was from 41 to 56. The corrected value from the Iraqi study (Bakir *et al.*, 1973) was 33 (and possibly as high as 41).

Converting Eq. (5) from blood to hair Hg using the ratio 0.367 that was found for this study results in:

$$\text{hair Hg (ug/L)} = 0.7 + 16 \text{ dietary intake (ug/kg/d)} \qquad (6)$$

which agrees reasonably well with hair/intake factors described above. Haxton *et al.* (1979) found a hair/blood ratio of 0.250; converting their blood/intake slopes to a hair basis yields hair/intake slopes of 10.5 and 12.2, also in reasonable agreement. The range of empirically determined hair/intake ratios thus appears to be from 10.5 to 16. However, studies whose underlying results are as poorly correlated as these do not allow determination of whether the underlying relationship is actually linear. Also, the range of blood/intake ratios appears to be proportionately wider than the range of blood/intake ratios, reflecting the variability in hair/blood ratios.

Kjellstrom *et al.*'s data (1986, 1989) on New Zealand mothers' exposure and children's IQ pose a more difficult analysis task. In this data set, 74 "cases" were identified from a cohort of 935, based on maternal hair > 6 ug/g and then matched with 163 controls having lower concentrations. The group-average hair Hg levels were 10.15 ug/g and 2.57 ug/g, respectively, but the frequencies of fish consumption were only slightly higher for the "cases". Both groups showed a tendency towards higher hair Hg with increasing fish consumption (Figure 5), but the intercepts

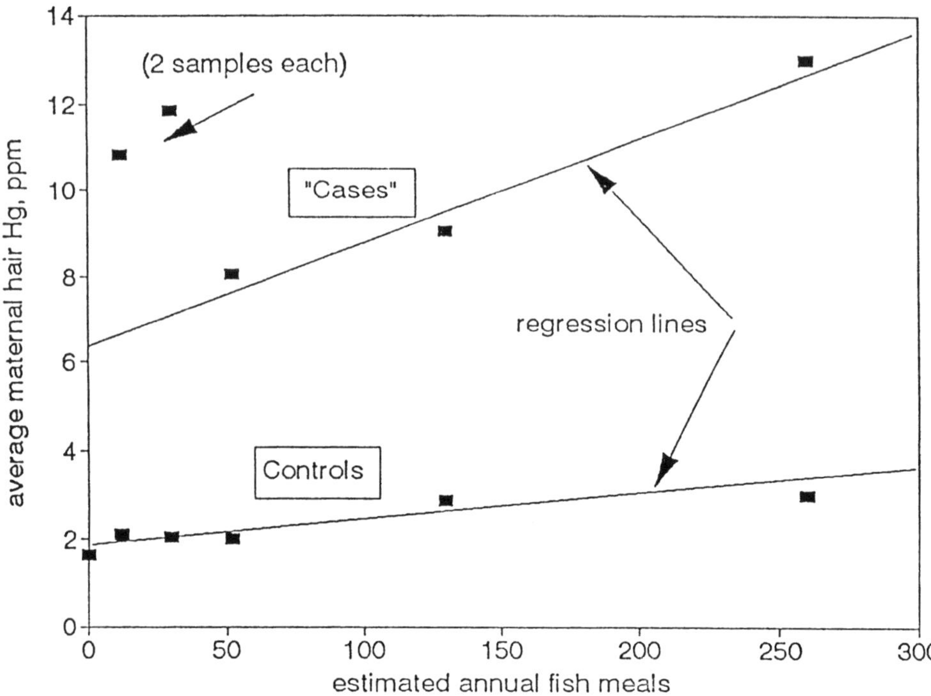

Fig. 5. Grouped-average hair concentrations vs. estimated MeHg intake from the data of Kjellstrom et al. (1989). "Cases" refer to the 73 individuals with the highest hair Hg concentrations; "controls" refer to others in the original cohort.

and slopes were quite different. Thus, use of an uncertain hair Hg value as a "case" selection criterion may have resulted in some misclassification (assuming reliable data on frequency of fish consumption). These results could be explained if the "cases" habitually consumed fish species with characteristically higher Hg content than the controls (by about a factor of 4). If an average fish Hg concentration of 0.24 ug/g is postulated for the "cases" and 0.06 ug/g for the controls (for the sake of illustration), the following relationships are derived that are approximately in line with those of other studies:

"cases": hair Hg = 6 + 10.5 intake (ug/kg/d) (7)

controls: hair Hg = 2 + 9.1 intake (ug/kg/d) (8)

The derived slope factors may be depressed because of the uncertainties in consumption measures or fish Hg content, but without independent estimates of the fish Hg content or meal size, this cannot be corroborated. Figure 5 and Eqs. (5) and (6) suggest that the measured hair values may be poor surrogates of actual exposure in this study because of the large difference in intercepts between the two subgroups (4 ug/g). The only logical explanations for this difference are either another source of Hg intake or else higher Hg concentration measurement errors for "cases". The results thus imply that only a portion of the higher hair Hg in the "cases" can be ascribed to MeHg intake, even if higher slopes were used to account for uncertainties in intake.

The relationship between dietary intake of Hg and hair or blood concentration might be more reliably portrayed by comparing population averages than individuals, since at least some of the uncertainties due to individual metabolic differences would be expected to average out. As an example, Airey (1983) presented the following empirical relationship based on data from 32 locations in 13 countries:

$$\text{Hair Hg (ug/g)} = 0.94 + 0.08 \text{ fish cons. (kg/pers/y)} + 0.47 \text{ GNP} \quad (\text{GNP in } 10^{12} \text{ \$US}) \quad (R=0.83)$$

Fish consumption accounted for 94% of the explained variance. Assuming that the world-wide average of Hg concentration in fish is 0.15 ug/g and that the average body mass is 60 kg yields a proportionality factor of 11.7, in reasonable agreement with the relationships derived above.

The blood/intake relationship used in the BNL risk assessment model (Lipfert et al., 1996) and given above is consistent with the controlled intake studies (which are more akin to laboratory than epidemiological studies) described by Sherlock and Quinn (1988) in which a 1 ug daily intake produces an equilibrium blood concentration of 0.8-1.0 ug/L in a 70 kg person. Sherlock and Quinn also attributed the findings by several uncontrolled (i.e., epidemiological) studies of substantially lower blood/intake slopes to the statistical effects of experimental error in the dietary intake data, as described above. However, after correcting for experimental error to the extent possible, the average ratio between equilibrium blood Hg and intake appears to be lower than expected by about 35%. This might be regarded as independent confirmation of a lower mean half-life for MeHg, in support of the recent findings of Smith and colleagues.

3.2 HAIR MERCURY vs. BLOOD MERCURY CONCENTRATIONS

Using hair concentration as an index of exposure to MeHg assumes a reasonably constant relationship between concentrations in hair and in other parts of the body (such as in blood), among the individuals involved. The statistical method used to estimate such relationships may be sensitive to measurement errors. If a linear regression is used, the slope (or its inverse) will be biased by uncertainty in the "independent" variable, as discussed above; the variable with the least uncertainty should be selected, even if this produces the reciprocal of the slope factor that is actually desired. Most investigators have used blood concentration as the independent variable. It is also possible to force the regression through the origin (Cernichiari *et al.*, 1995a), but this may not always be realistic at low concentrations, especially when total Hg rather than MeHg concentrations are used (there may be an intercept due to inorganic Hg in hair). A further alternative is to calculate the average of individual hair/blood ratios, but these can be unduly influenced by errors at low concentrations. As discussed below, Monte Carlo simulations were used to explore some of these problems.

Kazantzis *et al.* (1976) present some data on a large Iraqi cohort and noted that many of the blood samples were delayed substantially beyond the period of exposure, making it difficult to assess hair/blood ratios. Nevertheless, they report average ratios of 0.267 for unexposed subjects and 0.434 for those who ate contaminated bread. It seems likely that the latter value has been inflated by delayed blood sampling.

Equation (1) relates the blood concentration of MeHg to dietary intake rates; hair concentration is proportional to blood concentration but the constant of proportionality varies among individuals, just as the half-life required in Eq. (1) differs among individuals. Phelps *et al.* (1980) reported perhaps the best correlation between Hg in blood and in hair, from 340 residents of two Indian Reserve areas in northwestern Ontario that had eaten contaminated fish. Average concentrations were not reported, but the range appeared to be about 5 to 50 ug/g in hair. Atomic absorption analysis was used with bundles of about 100 strands for which longitudinal alignment had been preserved; the bundles were then cut into 1-cm segments for analysis. The blood-hair correlation presented was for the hair segments closest to the scalp (to correspond to the timing of blood sample collection):

$$\text{total Hg (hair, ug/g)} = 0.470 + 0.296 \text{ blood (ug/L)} \quad (R=0.935) \qquad (9)$$

$$\text{MeHg (hair, ug/g)} = 0.355 + 0.278 \text{ blood (ug/L)} \quad (R=0.940) \qquad (10)$$

The (implied) genetic similarity of this particular population, as well as the relatively high concentration levels (when compared to normal populations), may have contributed to the high blood/hair correlations found by Phelps *et al.*

From these data, measurement errors *per se* in blood or hair concentrations do not appear to be an issue when the sampling is appropriately timed. However, Eq. (10) is also consistent with a substantial variation in individual hair/blood ratios. As an illustration, the data of Phelps *et al.* were replicated *de novo* with a Monte Carlo simulation (n=340) starting with a log-normal distribution of blood Hg (GSD=2.0) and the normal distribution of hair/blood ratios (mean=0.267, sigma=0.067) that was used in the BNL simulation model (Lipfert *et al.*, 1996). The results are shown in Figure 6; the 95% confidence limits on the hair/blood ratio are approximately 0.19 and 0.33. However, in epidemiological practice, hair concentrations are more likely to be either averaged over the entire length of sample, or restricted to pregnancy, in which case the correlations with blood are likely to be attenuated. Phelps *et al.*'s data thus mainly verify the accuracy of measurement under idealized conditions.

Other hair-blood correlation coefficients using average hair concentrations tend to be lower, around 0.8. Hislop *et al.* (1983) found substantial variations in hair/blood ratios (from 0.200 to 0.340) among 5 volunteers fed identical fish diets for 3 months. Turner *et al.* (1980) derived relationships between hair and blood Hg for 140 Peruvian villagers:

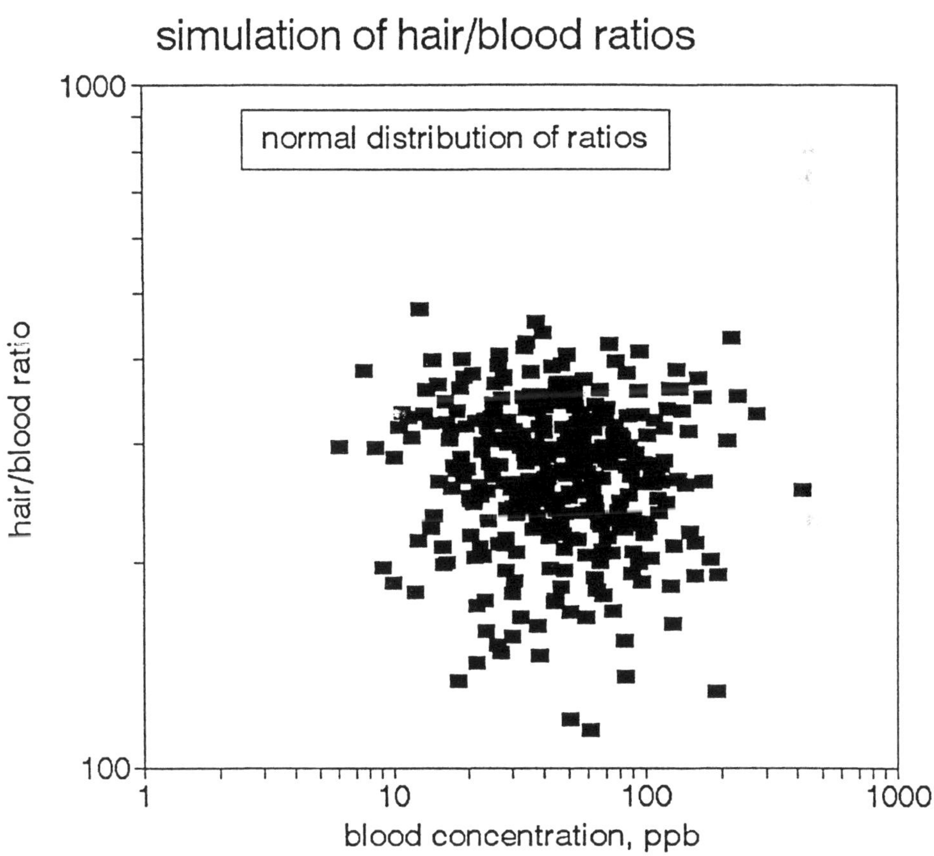

Fig. 6. Results from a Monte Carlo simulation of a typical range of variation in individual hair/blood concentration ratios, in the absence of measurement error.

for total Hg: hair Hg = 3.04 + 0.190 blood Hg (R=0.77)
for MeHg: hair MeHg = 0.47 + 0.191 blood MeHg (R=0.88)

These slopes would be higher (about 0.22-0.25) if the regressions were forced through the origin; most of the apparent outliers were in the direction of high hair values. In contrast, Sherlock *et al.* (1982) derived a very different relationship between total hair and blood Hg in the UK:

hair Hg = 0.694 + 0.367 blood Hg (n=98, R=0.84)

They found no improvement when organic Hg was used instead of total Hg. Since the correlation coefficients are similar in the Peruvian and English studies, it may be concluded that there may be bona fide differences in the hair-blood concentration relationship, even when averaged over population groups (perhaps due to ethnicity or hair color). However, the average of 0.190 and 0.367 (0.278) is very close to the overall average of hair-blood ratios used in the BNL model (0.267).

Skerfving (1974) found a hair/blood regression slope of 0.23, but this appears to be highly dependent on two high-Hg individuals that had reduced their intakes of MeHg before blood sampling. Thus, hair and blood samples are incompatible for these two observations; deleting them would reduce the slope to about 0.16. In addition, these data are for blood cells rather than whole blood, a fact that seems to have been overlooked by both WHO (1990) and ATSDR (1994) in citing Skerfving's results. Correcting by the ratio of 0.54 (see Eq. 3) yields a hair/blood slope of 0.30, which is in line with expectations.

For the Faroe Island study, Dahl *et al.* (1996) reported mean hair and blood concentrations of 4.5 ug/g and 24.2 ng/L, which implies a mean ratio of about 0.19. The correlation was not given.

The Seychelles Island Study (Cernichiari *et al.*, 1995a) reported an average hair/blood ratio of 0.416. For this group of 27 mothers, this average value is outside the expected range discussed above. However, it was obtained by regressing blood concentration on hair concentration, thus placing the least certain variable as the independent variable. Since these regressions were forced through the origin, interpreting the results is less straightforward and thus Monte Carlo simulations were used as a guide. These showed that assuming the normal range of hair-blood ratios for a group of 27 individuals could not produce the results reported by Cernichiari *et al.* (R=0.82, blood/hair slope=2.4, std. err.=0.2) when forced through the origin, unless extraneous measurement error was added to the system. Without the error, the correlations were much higher than Cernichiari *et al.* reported, similar to the results of Phelps *et al.* (1980). The only alternative explanation would be that the true hair/blood ratios of this cohort lie outside the expected range obtained from many other sources, which would imply that the Seychelles study population differs from others.

Grandjean et al. (1992) report similar findings with respect to the relationship between maternal hair and cord blood, for about 1000 Faroe Island women. They report a slope of 0.11 with hair Hg as the dependent variable (apparently not forced through the origin), and 4.8 (corresponding to an inverse slope of 0.21) with blood Hg as the dependent variable. The correlation coefficient implied by these two values is about 0.73, and the sampling uncertainties are quite small because of the large cohort. Thus the major uncertainty is the source of the errors that reduce the correlation below 1.0.

Finally, the source of the errors that drive correlations between hair and blood below the "ideal" reported by Phelps *et al.* (1980) may not always be clear. Sampling errors in hair may be responsible (due to heterogeneity on the head) but, alternatively, blood samples may not reflect the same long-term average as the hair samples because of recent MeHg ingestion. This source of disagreement will tend to be emphasized for those consuming fish infrequently, *i.e.*, for low exposures.

4. Effects of Measurement Error in "Case" Selection

The study of IQ-Hg relationships in New Zealand children by Kjellstrom *et al.* (1986, 1989) began with a cohort of 11,000 births to mothers who completed a dietary intake survey. A set of 935 that reported frequent fish consumption was then tested for hair Hg concentrations, from which a subset of 74 suspected "cases" (of Hg effects on childhood development) was selected. The question arises as to what extent errors in measurement might have misclassified these "cases." Because there were no other direct exposure measurements, Monte Carlo simulations were used to re-create the data required to estimate the potential effects of measurement errors, assuming that theoretical distributions may be used for this purpose. The underlying hypothesis here is that selecting the highest observed hair concentrations may also select the largest measurement errors (recall that "error" as used here includes individual variability).

Whereas the traditional case-control methodology uses an outcome variable to select "cases", Kjellstrom *et al.* used a descriptive variable, the Hg content of maternal hair. They selected 74 "cases" having hair Hg concentrations in excess of 6 ug/g and 163 "controls" having lower hair Hg that were selected to match other characteristics of the "cases". The mean hair Hg concentrations of the two subsets were 10.15 and 2.57 ug/g, respectively. Monte Carlo simulations were used to investigate the likely properties of such a dataset; a lognormal distribution of blood Hg and a normal distribution of hair/blood ratios were used to generate an expected set of 935 hair concentrations. A distribution of random errors (mean=zero) was then added to these hair values using a multiplicative factor (to preclude negative concentrations and as suggested by the data of Airey *et al.*, 1983) to simulate the actual hair measurements that Kjellstrom *et al.* used. The distributions were tailored to produce about 7% of the hair values in excess of 6 ug/g (as found in the NZ data) and a maternal blood-hair correlation around 0.75, which is typical of many studies. Without the additional hair measurement error, this correlation was 0.94, similar to that found by Phelps *et al.* (1980) based on the hair segment next to the scalp. The additional hair measurement error included in the simulation was thus intended to represent uncertainties in locating the peak hair Hg concentration during pregnancy and the appropriate timing of exposure relative to fetal development.

The simulated "controls" were selected randomly from the remaining hair values in excess of 0.5 ug/g, which was the minimum value reported by Kjellstrom *et al.* (probably because of instrumental detection limits). However, the simulated control group had lower hair Hg values than were reported by Kjellstrom *et al.*, probably because the cohort of 935 births had been selected on the basis of reported above-average fish consumption.

Three Hg concentration variables, assumed to be steady in time, are of interest here: maternal blood Hg (which is hypothesized to represent the potential for prenatal exposure of the infant), maternal hair Hg as measured, and maternal hair Hg without measurement error but reflecting the expected distribution of individual hair/blood ratios (defined here as the "true" maternal hair Hg concentration). There are three subgroups of interest: the entire simulation data set (n=935), the high hair Hg subset (n=74), and the entire dataset considered by Kjellstrom *et al.* (n=237). Table I presents the relevant correlations produced by a single realization of this simulation:

Table I Hg Correlations Produced by NZ Data Simulations

	n=935		n=237		n=74	
hair data:	meas.	true	meas.	true	meas.	true
blood corr.	0.73	0.94	0.80	0.95	0.56	0.88
hair corr.	1.0	0.78	1.0	0.85	1.0	0.67

In each dataset, the correlation between measured and "true" hair concentrations is a good predictor of the measurement-error degradation of the hair-blood correlation (as expected), and presumably, also of any adverse health effects that would be predicted by the maternal blood concentration.

The mean hair/blood ratio for the "cases" was 0.473 with the additional error and 0.298 without it; this implies an average upward bias in hair Hg of about 60% from using a flawed measurement to select "cases". The mean "true" hair/blood ratio is also higher than the overall average (0.27), showing that the "case" selection process tends to pick out the (naturally) high hair/blood ratios as well as the indicated high Hg concentrations. A regression of "measured" hair concentration on blood concentration for the highest 74 hair observations yielded:

$$\text{hair Hg} = 3.45 + 0.261 \text{ blood Hg} \tag{11}$$

suggesting an average bias in the high-end hair measurements of about 3.45 ug/g, which is a substantial fraction of the original "case" selection criterion and checks well with Figure 6. These problems are most severe at the extremes of the distribution of measured hair concentrations; the correlation between the "true" and "measured" hair estimates for all 237 observations was 0.85 but the correlation between the 74 highest values with and without the additional error was 0.67. This means that a negative bias of about 50% (R^2) would be introduced into any dose-response functions (DRFs) based on that subset of hair measurements. In addition, the uncertainty about the true maternal hair Hg concentration and the corresponding infant brain Hg concentration would have furthered the downward bias on DRF slopes and intercepts. With these two important uncertainties in the exposure variable, it should not be surprising to encounter difficulty in determining the presence of adverse Hg effects.

In designing their study, Kjellstrom *et al.* intended to select the 74 births most likely to exhibit adverse effects of maternal Hg intake. However, such a selection process may not be appropriate in the presence of measurement error, because the probability of misclassification increases with the magnitude of the selection variable (with multiplicative errors). In other words, many of the 74 "cases" may have been selected because of high errors rather than because of high Hg exposures. Only 29 of the 74 "cases" had "true" hair values above 6 ug/g in this simulation, and the true maximum value was 19 rather than 40 ug/g. It would have been better to work with the entire cohort of 935 births; since these data are not available, the next best procedure is probably to pool Kjellstrom *et al.*'s "cases" and "controls" for analysis.

5. Use of Population-Average Exposure Metrics

When large populations are used, it is difficult to obtain reliable dietary intake information, even though the population statistics may be estimated reasonably well, especially in the long term. Hence, epidemiological studies employing individual dietary intake as an exposure measure will inevitably underestimate the relationships. According to Rose (1990), it is reasonable to expect similar distributions within populations, so that aggregating individuals into groups may remove some of this intra-individual variation and produce more reliable statistics.

Figure 7 compares population average (or median) hair Hg concentrations and dietary intake rates for fish-eating populations, from the epidemiological literature. Many of the dietary intake data had to be estimated from assumed meal sizes and estimates of the mean fish Hg consumed; Table II gives these details.

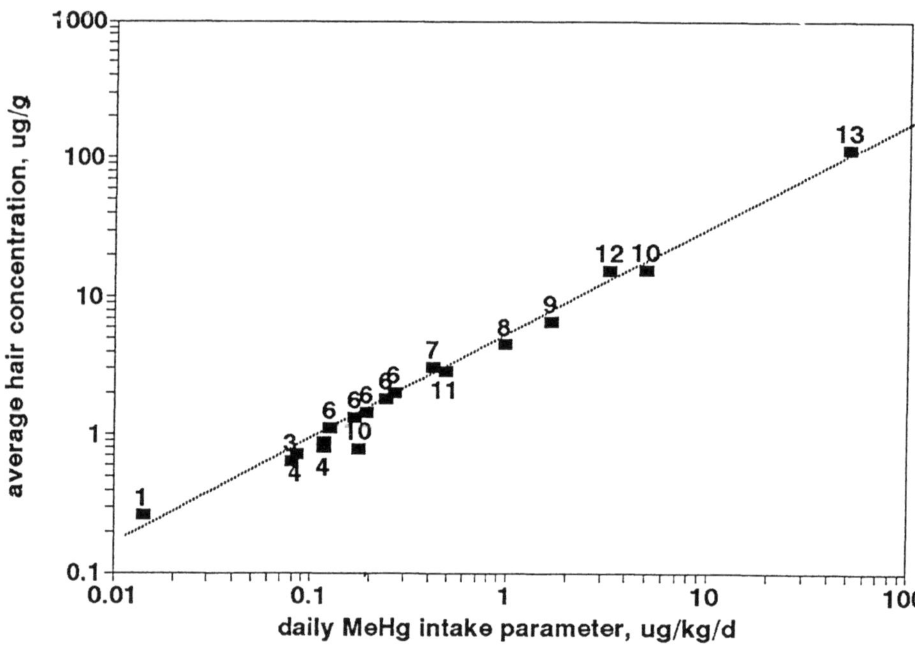

Fig. 7. Relationship between average hair Hg concentrations from various epidemiological studies of fish-eating populations and their respective average Hg dietary intake rates. See Table II for identification of the numbered data points.

Table II Population-averaged hair Hg and dietary intake data

graph ID	location	meals/wk	meal size g	fish Hg ug/g	intake ug/d	body mass,kg	intake ug/kg/d	hair Hg ug/g	hair/intake ratio	remarks	reference
1	all U.S.				1.0	70	0.014	0.26	18.20	1	Smith et al., 1985
3	S. Ontarlo						0.079	0.63	7.97	1	S. Paradis, pers. commumication
4	St Regis reservation				5.9	70	0.084	0.72	8.54	1	Valciukas et al., 1986
4	St Regis reservation				8.1	70	0.116	0.86	7.42	1	Valciukas et al., 1986
4	St Regis reservation				8.2	70	0.117	0.79	6.74	1	Valciukas et al., 1986
6	UK				18.6	70	0.265	2	7.54		Haxton et al., 1979
6	UK				13.4	70	0.192	1.43	7.45		Haxton et al., 1979
6	UK				16.9	70	0.241	1.8	7.47		Haxton et al., 1979
6	UK				8.7	70	0.124	1.1	8.84		Haxton et al., 1979
6	UK				11.7	70	0.167	1.31	7.83		Haxton et al., 1979
7	NZ	2.2	200	0.4	25.2	60	0.420	3.1	7.38		Kjellstrom et al., 1989
8	Faroe Is.				67.7	70	0.968	4.5	4.65	2	Grandjean et al., 1992
9	Seychelle Is.	12	200	0.289	99.1	60	1.651	6.6	4.00		Cernichiari et al., 1995
10	Peru				8.8	50	0.175	0.78	4.45	3	Turner et al., 1980
10	Peru			1.06	246.7	50	4.934	15.58	3.16	4	Turner et al., 1980
11	Amazon	1.69	200	0.5	24.1	50	0.483	2.87	5.94		Grandjean et al., 1993
13	Minamata, Japan	7	200	15	3000	60	50.000	115	2.30	5	Tsubaki & Irukayama, 1977
12	New Guinea	14.0	200	0.49	196	60	3.267	15.50	4.74		Kyle & Ghani, 1982

1. intake provided directly
2. based on whale & fish total
3. 1.9 kg/wk for 6.2 people
4. 10.1 kg/wk for 6.2 people
5. hair Hg estimated

The range of intake rates covers almost four orders of magnitude in intake but only three orders in hair concentrations; the characteristic slope appears to be an approximately 3/4 power relationship that is significantly lower than unity. A log-log regression provided an estimate of the slope of 0.77 with a standard error of 0.025 and an R^2 of 0.984.

At low intake rates, hair Hg is about 15 times daily intake (as expected), but at the highest rates the ratio approaches 2.0. However, the estimates for Minimata may be problematic: a daily 200 g meal at 15 ppm was assumed. An estimate of the median hair concentration was scaled from the maximum reported value, 705 ppm. This sub-linear trend is not predicted by theory and cannot be attributed to uncertainties in dietary distributions at high doses since the Monte Carlo simulation and Figure 4 suggested that dietary variability was greatest at low (infrequent) intake rates. Note that the overall trend of Figure 7 is not dependent upon the data from any one study nor is it dependent upon assumptions about meal size or body mass.

6. Conclusions

This review and analysis has shown that at least some of the conventional wisdom in the literature on MeHg dose-response relationships has been biased by the effects of uncertainties in exposures. While some of the published relationships between blood concentration and intake seem to have been affected by intake measurement error, as a group and after adjusting for such errors, they support a lower half-life for MeHg, consistent with recent findings of Smith and colleagues (1994, 1996). This suggests that realistic analyses of health risks should be based on the lower half-life figures. Our previous risk analyses (Lipfert *et al.*, 1994, 1996) may thus represent overestimates.

Most studies of the effects of prenatal exposures to MeHg have relied on maternal hair concentrations as a surrogate for fetal exposures, which implies essentially constant ratios of MeHg concentrations in the various physiological "compartments" involved, for each population. However, considerable differences exist among individuals in terms of hair/blood Hg concentration ratios. This does not preclude a high correlation between the two measures under carefully controlled conditions. However, individuals may exhibit higher (or lower) hair Hg concentrations than expected from their true exposure to dietary Hg simply because of this source of intra-individual random variation. Thus, large populations may be required for reliable epidemiological results. When average hair Hg and dietary intake rates are compared across studies of fish-eating populations, a nonlinear relationship becomes apparent, implying that higher intakes of MeHg do not result in proportionately higher hair concentrations. This phenomenon should be investigated further before any specific study is used as the basis for setting dietary intake standards for fish of MeHg.

If the varying population-average hair/blood ratios are indeed real, the use of hair concentration as the epidemiological metric of choice becomes problematic. Given a valid-dose response function based on hair concentrations, a population with hair/blood ratios higher than average may inappropriately be considered at risk, and vice-versa. A particularly variable early set of hair Hg data was obtained from "non-exposed" individuals in Iraq that leads to suspicions of excessive errors in measurement, usually on the high side.

The available measures of adult exposures to MeHg compare reasonably well with one another when these uncertainties are taken into account. However, the exposures of infants *in utero* will inevitably be less certain than those of the mothers; thus, bias is to be expected in prenatal dose-response functions based on maternal hair concentrations. Those biases will underestimate the slope and will shift any apparent intercepts towards the left. This important source of bias must be considered when comparing the relative sensitivities of adults with infants that have been prenatally exposed to methylmercury.

In view of the importance of obtaining accurate exposure measures in epidemiology, investigators are urged to obtain (and present) data on more than one exposure metric, so that their relative uncertainties may be assessed independently. In addition, the development of more reliable methods of assessing dietary intake should be considered for future epidemiological studies.

Acknowledgments

Most of this research was supported by the U.S. Department of Energy, Office of Clean Coal Technology; Dr. Lawrence Saroff was the Project Officer. No official endorsement should be inferred. The helpful comments of two reviewers are gratefully acknowledged. This paper was originally edited by Dr. Avril Woodhead.

References

Agency for Toxic Substances and Disease Registry (ATSDR): 1994, Toxicological Profile for Mercury (update), U.S. Dept. Health & Human Services, Atlanta, GA.

Airey, D.: 1983, *Environ.Health Perspect.* **52**, 303-16.

Al-Shahristani, H., and Shihab, K.: 1974, *Arch.Environ.Health* **28**, 342-4.

Al-Shahristani, H., Shihab, K., and Al-Haddad, I.K.: 1976, *Conference on Intoxication Due to Alklymercury-Treated Seed*, Baghdad, WHO, Geneva, pp. 105-11.

Al-Shahristani, H., and Al-Haddad, I.K.: 1973, *J.Radioanal.Chem.* **15**, 59-70.

Bakir, F., *et al.*: 1973, *Science* **181**, 230-241.

Birke, G. *et al.*: 1972, *Arch.Environ.Health* **25**, 77-91.

Cernichiari, E., *et al.*: 1995a, *NeuroToxicology* **16**, 705-11.

Cernichiari, E., *et al.*: 1995b, *NeuroToxicology* **16**, 613-28.

Eads, E.E., and Lambdin, C.E.: 1973, *Envir.Res.* **6**, 247-52.

Englender, S.J., Landrigan, P.J., Greenwood, M.R., Atwood, R.G., Clarkson, T.W., and Smith, J.C.: 1980, *Arch.Envir.Health* **35**, 224-8.

Grandjean, P. *et al.*: 1992, *Arch.Environ.Health* **47**, 185-95.

Grandjean, P., Cardoso, B., and Guimaraes, G.: 1993, *Lancet* **342**, 991.

Grandjean, P., Weihe, P., and White, R.F.: 1995, *NeuroToxicology* **16**, 27-34.

Haxton, J. *et al.*: 1979, *Envir. Res.* **18**, 351-68.

Hislop, J.S., Collier, T.R., White, G.F., Khathing, D.T., and French, E.: 1983, *Chemical Toxicology and Clinical Chemistry of Metals*, ed. by S. Brown and J. Savory, Academic Press, London, 1983. pp. 145-8.

Kazantzis, G. *et al.*: 1976, *Conference on Intoxication Due to Alklymercury-Treated Seed*, Baghdad, Iraq, WHO, Geneva.

Kjellstrom, T., Kennedy, P., Wallis, S., and Mantell, C.: Physical and Mental Development of Children with Prenatal Exposure to Mercury from Fish. Stage 1: Preliminary Tests at Age 4. Report 3080, National Swedish Environmental Protection Board, Solna, Sweden, 1986.

Kjellstrom, T., Kennedy, P., Wallis, S., Stewart, A., Friburg, L., Lind, B., Wutherspoon, T. and Mantell, C.: Physical and Mental Development of Children with Prenatal Exposure to Mercury from Fish. Stage 2: Interviews and Psychological Tests at Age 6. Report 3642, National Swedish Environmental Protection Board, Solna, Sweden, 1989.

Kyle, J.H., and Ghani, N.: 1982, *Arch.Envir.Health* **37**, 266-70.

Lipfert, F., Moskowitz, P., Fthenakis, V., DePhillips, M., Viren, J., and Saroff, L.: 1994, Assessment of Mercury Health Risks to Adults from Coal Combustion, BNL-60435, Brookhaven National Laboratory, Upton, NY.

Lipfert, F., Moskowitz, P., Fthenakis, V., DePhillips, M., Viren, J., Saroff, L.: 1996, *NeuroToxicology* **17**, 197-211.

Marsh, D.O., *et al.*: 1987, *Arch.Neurol.* **44**, 1017-22.

Marsh, D.O., Turner, M.D., Smith, J.C., Allen, P., and Richdale, N.: 1995, *NeuroToxicology* **16**, 717-26.

Miettinen, J.K.: 1972, *Mercury, Mercurials, and Mercaptans*, ed. by M.W. Miller and T.W. Clarkson, Thomas, Springfield, IL, 1972, pp. 233-43.

Phelps, R.W., Clarkson, T.W., Kershaw, T.G., and Wheatley, B.: 1980, *Arch.Env.Health* **35**, 161-8

Rose, G., and Day, S.: 1990, *Brit.Med.J.* **301**, 1031-4.

Sherlock, J.C., and Quinn, M.J.: 1988, *Human Toxicol.* **7**, 129-32.

Sherlock, J.C., *et al.*: 1982, *Arch.Env.Health* **37**, 271-8.

Shimomura, S., Kimura, A., Nakagawa, H., and Takao, M.: 1980, *Envir.Res.* **22**, 22-30.

Skerfving, S.: 1974, *Toxicology* **2**, 3-23.

Sky-Peck, H.H., and Joseph, B.L.: 1983, *Chemical Toxicology and Clinical Chemistry of Metals*, ed. by S.S. Brown and J. Savory, Academic Press, London, pp. 159-63.

Smith, J.C., Turner ,M.D., and Marsh, D.O.: 1985, *Report on Project III* to National Fisheries Institute.

Smith, J.C., Allen, P., Turner, M., Most, B., Fisher, H.L., and Hall, L.L.: 1994, *Toxicol. Appl. Pharmacol.* **128**, 251-6.

Smith, J.C., and Farris, F.F.: 1996, *Toxicol. Appl. Pharmacol.* **137**, 245-52.

Spitzer, W.O., *et al.*: 1988, *Clin.Invest.Med.* **11**, 71-97.

Thomas, D., Stram, D., and Dwyer, J.: 1993, *Ann.Rev.Public Health* **14**, 69-93.

Tsubaki, T., and Irukayama, K., ed.: 1977, *Minamata Disease*, Elsevier, Amsterdam.

Turner, M.D., *et al.*: 1980, *Arch.Env.Health* **35**, 367-78.

Valciukas, J.A., Levin, S.M., Nicholson, W.J., and Selikoff, I.J.: 1986, *Arch.Env.Health* **41**, 269-72.

World Health Organization (WHO): 1990, *Methylmercury*, Environmental Health Criteria 101, Geneva, 144 pp.

Mercury Contamination Through Fish Consumption: A Model for Predicting and Preventing Hazardous Behaviour on a Community Level.

Sylvain Paradis[1], Brian Wheatley[1], Jane Boswell-Purdy[1], Denis Bélisle[2], Maxine Cole[3], Henry Lickers[4], Alan Hayton[5], and Kate Davies[6]

[1]*Research & Development, Environmental Contaminants, Medical Services Branch, Health Canada, Jeanne Mance Bldg. Rm, 1170, P. L. 1911D, Tunney's Pasture, Ottawa, Ontario, K1A 0L3, Canada.* [2]*Département de Psychologie, Faculté des Lettres et Sciences Humaines, Université de Sherbrooke, Sherbrooke, Québec, Canada.* [3]*EAGLE Project Coordinating Office, Assembly of First Nations, 1 Nicholas St., Ottawa, Ontario, K1N 7B7, Canada.* [4]*Mohawk Council of Akwesasne, P.O. Box 579, Cornwall, Ontario, K6H 5T3, Canada.* [5]*Ontario Ministry of Environment and Energy, 125 Resources Road, Rexdale, Ontario, M9P 3V6, Canada.* [6]*Ecosystems Consulting Inc., 2151 Fillmore Crescent, Gloucester, Ontario, K1J 6A1, Canada*

Abstract. The relationship between the consumption of fish containing methylmercury (MeHg) and human MeHg levels has been studied for many years. Although this relationship has been demonstrated and some models have been developed to assess the risks associated with fish consumption, there is still a need for a simple and efficient predicting tool that can be applied to community settings. This paper provides such a practical model developed through empirical evidence using two sources of data.

In ideal conditions, models used to identify hazardous behaviour in individuals would be derived from theoretical and clinical models, however, these conditions are often technically difficult to meet. To overcome this problem, a more empirically oriented model has been developed, based on the estimation of personal mercury intake and its comparison to the Tolerable Daily Intake. The theory and methodology of the model development, including technical limitations, are presented first. The methodology is then applied to the real data to create the final model and the results given. Finally, a discussion of the model's accuracy, limitations and usefulness as a community health assessment tool is presented.

1. Introduction

The relationship between the consumption of fish containing methylmercury (MeHg), and human exposure to MeHg (WHO, 1990) through fish consumption has been documented by various researchers. Although some models have been developed to assess the risks associated with the consumption of fish containing mercury (Birke *et al*., 1972), there is still a need for simple, predictive models which can be applied to community settings. The purpose of this paper is to describe a method by which individuals can estimate whether their mercury intake is above the Tolerable Daily Intake (TDI) by keeping track of the frequency and size of fish meals consumed.

There are a variety of models currently used to associate fish consumption and contaminant intake. One of the most common methods is to link fish consumption directly to contaminant levels in blood or hair. In this type of model contaminants in fish are often not established, using frequency of consumption as the sole measure of intake (Hovinga *et al*, 1993 and Fleming *et al*, 1995). In other studies, fish levels have been measured but for only one or two species (Birke *et al*, 1972 and Kyle and Ghani, 1982). In either situation, assumptions, rather than actual values, are usually used for important factors such as meal size and personal body weight, or ignored completely. Another type of model relies only on fish contaminant levels, excluding personal data entirely (using assumed levels of consumption, meal size and body weight) to produce consumption advisories, such as those released by the Ontario Ministry of Environment and Energy (MOEE, 1995).

In Canada, research on human exposure to mercury has focused largely on the country's aboriginal population (Wheatley and Paradis, 1995, 1996). With higher fish consumption and average body weight than the general population (EAGLE, 1996a), and a reliance on the freshwater fish supply for subsistence, members of Canada's First Nations are at greater risk for exposure to mercury in fish. For the past five years, the EAGLE (Effects on Aboriginals from the Great Lakes Environment) Project, a partnership between First Nations in the Great Lakes Basin, the Assembly of First Nations and Health Canada has been examining First Nations' exposure to mercury and other environmental contaminants in fish as part of its mandate to document and understand the effects of environmental contaminants on human health. The first component of the EAGLE Fish Contaminants Program was to assess the availability of information on contaminants in fish from locations close to the participating First Nations communities. This assessment was then used as a basis for deciding where additional fish samples were needed. The second component was to produce fish consumption guidelines for each of the communities. Finally, individuals displaying potentially hazardous behaviour relative to mercury intake were identified, on the basis of their fish consumption. This paper focusses on the third component only.

A related program within EAGLE, its Eating Patterns Survey (EPS), provided data on fish consumption and demographics that were used in this study. Levels of mercury in freshwater fish were obtained from the Ontario Ministry of Environment and Energy which regularly conducts tests on samples collected from the Great Lakes Basin. These data have also been used to study the effects of acidic deposition on areas known to have high mercury levels (Richardson *et al*, 1993). Richardson established several factors that influence the levels of mercury in fish including the lake, fish species, the fish length (as a measure of age) and the type of contaminant. These factors have been taken into account in this study.

To develop a model to identify hazardous behaviour in individuals, mercury levels in fish and data from the EPS, were combined and compared with the TDI for methylmercury of 0.47 μg/kg body weight per day (WHO, 1990). With TDI expressed as the number of micrograms of contaminant per kilogram of body weight per day (μg/kgbw/day), similarly an actual daily intake can be calculated from the level of a contaminant present in the fish consumed and the amount consumed. By calculating an average level of mercury in the fish for each community and individual average daily fish consumption per kg body weight, a Personal Daily Intake (PDI) of mercury for each individual in a community can be estimated. This PDI is then compared to the known TDI to identify people who may be exposed to amounts of mercury in excess of the TDI. Having identified these individuals whose behaviour may pose a hazard to their health, further analysis was carried out to determine which factors, if any, distinguish these consumers from those with low PDIs. Knowledge of these distinguishing factors provides a basis for the simple model created to predict potentially hazardous behaviour.

The model presented here is different from those mentioned above for a number of reasons. Rather than measuring the end result of mercury intake through hair or blood, we have attempted to estimate the actual ingestion levels at the front end of the process. We have based our estimates on a much larger database of fish contaminant levels, covering a larger number of species. The direct integration of TDI into the model appears to be unique to our model. Real data concerning meal sizes and body weights make it possible to apply the model on an individual basis while still being able to expand the method to the overall target population. The main innovation with this model lies in its ability to empower the individual to judge his/her own relative hazard. He/she does not have to worry about keeping track of specific advisories associated with different species or sites; these factors have been directly incorporated into the model. Individuals will be given a simple tool to determine for themselves a safe pattern of fish consumption. Further details concerning the limitations, purpose and target population of the model will be discussed in a separate EAGLE document (EAGLE, 1996b).

2. Methodology

2.1 THE DATA

The data used in the analysis were taken from two main sources. For the estimation of mercury levels in the fish, data were made available by the MOEE. Demographic information and individual fish consumption data were extracted from the EPS. The information contained in each data file, in combination with the other, dictated the final dataset used in the analysis. The various data elements taken from each source, and the selection procedures and criteria applied to those data are discussed below.

The EPS provided data for a total of 1486 individuals in 30 First Nation communities, surveyed between 1993 and 1995. A number of different criteria had to be met for individual cases to remain in the analysis. The results of the survey showed that the 6 most commonly eaten species (based on total weight consumed yearly) are pickerel (*Stizostedion vitreum*), whitefish (*Coregonus clupeaformis*), northern pike (*Esox lucius*), lake trout (*Salvelinus namaycush*), bass (*Micropterus dolomieui* and *Micropterus salmoides*) and perch (*Perca flavescens*). It was decided to limit the analysis to these 6 species only, and the individuals who consumed them because these six species account for 76% of all fish consumed. Furthermore, because PDI estimates are a function of individual body weight and community specific mercury levels, anyone for whom this information was not available had to be excluded from the analysis. Close examination of the EPS data revealed some individuals with levels of fish consumption (in terms of meal size) in the extreme of the high end of the distribution. It is believed that these cases do not accurately represent the central body of the population for which the final model was being developed. It was therefore decided to remove these consumption outliers. The method used to identify and eliminate the outliers was that of a boxplot of the consumption distribution. Males tend to consume larger quantities of fish than females and consequently the distribution was considered separately for each gender. The variable of interest was the average fish-meal weight (over the 6 species) in grams. A boxplot of the variable was constructed and all individuals falling outside the upper limit of

$$75\text{th percentile} + 1.5\times\text{IQR}$$

where $\text{IQR} = \text{Interquartile Range} = 75\text{th percentile} - 25\text{th percentile}$,

were removed from the dataset. The final sample population used for the analysis consisted of 880 EPS respondents.

Reason for Removal	# of Cases Removed	% of 1486	# of Cases Remaining
Did not consume fish	262	17.63	1224
Did not consume 6 species of interest	62	4.17	1162
Missing body weight	38	2.56	1124
No mercury levels	171	11.51	953
Consumption outlier	73	4.91	880
Total	**606**	**40.78**	**880**

Table I Removal of EPS cases, from n=1486 to n=880

The original MOEE data provided test results for 61 different contaminants in 59 species of fish, taken from 641 sampling sites. The samples were collected over a 17 year period from 1978 to 1994. The data contained a total of 487,557 observations, each representing a single contaminant test performed on a particular fish from a specific sampling site. For our purposes, the number of observations was reduced in this dataset also.

It was decided to consider only the previous ten years of data on mercury levels in fish, i.e., 1984 - 1994 because older data are unlikely to be indicative of current mercury levels and because they are less likely to be reliable than more recent data. Where species from the same site had been re-sampled within the last ten years, the most recent data were used.

Results of the EPS showed that community members tended to fish within a radius of approximately 25 kilometres of their community. Their actual fishing sites were recorded by latitude and longitude and checked against sampled sites in the MOEE data and seven additional sites sampled by members of the communities through the EAGLE project. The analysis used mercury data from community relevant sampled sites only.

Approximately 86% of the fish reported to be eaten by EPS respondents was "skinless, boneless fillets". Furthermore, 89.1% of all MOEE analyses were conducted on this portion of the fish. For comparability of test results and relevance to the target population, only data on these samples were selected for use.

A subset of the MOEE fish contaminant data was selected using the criteria outlined above. This subset was used to estimate average mercury levels for each fishing site-species subgroup. To do this, a knowledge of the relationship between fish length and the measured mercury concentrations is necessary. This meant that observations with missing mercury levels or fish lengths were eliminated, as were those from all site-species subgroups with less than 10 complete observations.

2.2 ESTIMATING COMMUNITY-SPECIFIC MERCURY LEVELS

Before estimating personal mercury intake it was necessary to predict mercury levels for the fish likely to be consumed by that person. This meant that levels were estimated for each community separately.

As mentioned above, fish length was used as the sole predictor of site-specific mercury levels in the fish, the rationale being that mercury levels increase with age, with length being used as a surrogate measure of a fish's age. The form of the relationship used was a non-linear one suggested by the literature (Ricker, 1979). For each community *i*, site *j*, species *k* subgroup, a power regression was performed to determine the relationship between mercury level and fish length for that subgroup, and the regression coefficients saved for later use:

$$level = X_{ijk} * length^{Y_{ijk}}$$

As the lengths of the actual fish eaten by the EPS respondents were not known, it was necessary to use some type of standard length when estimating the average mercury level for any given species within a community. It was decided to use a length representative of what might be considered a "big" fish. Given the relationship between the relative mercury level and fish length, use of the "big" fish will result in a more cautious estimate of the PDI. The definition of a "big" fish would depend upon the usual length of fish sampled (caught) in that community. Therefore, for each species, *k*, sampled within community *i*, the mean length (over all community sampling sites) was calculated. A "big" fish was then considered to be 1 standard deviation larger than the mean:

$$big_{ik} = \underset{j}{\text{mean}}(length_{ik}) + \underset{j}{\text{sd}}(length_{ik})$$

This length was then used in the non-linear relationship above (using the previously determined regression coefficients) to calculate the average mercury level in species *k*, from site *j* in community *i*, for a "big" fish:

$$level_{ijk} = X_{ijk} * big_{ik}^{Y_{ijk}}$$

Next, an overall average mercury level/loading (over all community sites) was calculated for each species within a community, as

$$load_{ik} = \underset{j}{\text{mean}}(level_{ijk})$$

This was the quantity used in the personal intake model described below.

2.3 PREDICTING PERSONAL MERCURY INTAKE

With personal data available from the EPS, and community-specific mercury level estimates computed, it was possible to identify individuals with a possibly high level of mercury intake. For each member, *m*, of a community, *i*, a PDI was calculated for mercury. Since mercury levels are species dependant, intake must first be calculated separately for each species, *k*, eaten by the individual as:

$$pdi_{mik} = \frac{(total_{mik} * load_{ik})/365}{weight_{mi}} \qquad k = 1, \ldots, 6$$

where

pdi_{mik} = portion of total personal daily intake of mercury for person *m* of community *i* (PDI_{mi}) attributed to species *k*, in μg/kgbw/day

$total_{mik}$ = total yearly consumption of species k, in grams (may be 0), for person m of community i

$load_{ik}$ = average mercury loading (level) for species k (for size "big"), over all locations for community i, in μg/g

$weight_{mi}$ = body weight, in kg for person m of community i

All individual species-specific *pdi*'s were then summed over all species, to get a total PDI for that individual,

$$\mathrm{PDI}_{mi} = \sum_{k=1}^{6} pdi_{mik}$$

The estimated daily intake of mercury was then compared to the TDI for methylmercury, to determine whether that individual's consumption constitutes hazardous behaviour; i.e.

$$\mathrm{PDI}_{mi} > \mathrm{TDI} \Rightarrow \text{person } m \text{ may be ingesting too much mercury}$$

This comparison assumes that an individual's entire daily intake of methylmercury comes from fish consumption. In fact, the World Health Organization attributes virtually 100% (2.4 μg/day of a total 2.41 μg/day) of all methylmercury intake to fish consumption (WHO, 1990). Therefore, we have allocated the full TDI of 0.47 μg/kgbw/day to fish consumption for the purposes of the comparison above.

This process resulted in estimates of mercury PDIs for each of the 880 individuals.

2.4 A MODEL FOR IDENTIFYING HAZARDOUS INDIVIDUAL CONSUMPTION PATTERNS

The estimated personal mercury intake levels (as calculated in this analysis) are a function of a number of factors, including the type of species eaten, the amount of each species eaten and the relative amount of contamination in those species. However, it was the goal of this analysis to provide a simple model which individuals in the study communities could apply to their own consumption habits to prevent themselves from possible hazardous exposure to mercury through fish consumption. The task was therefore to simplify the function as much as possible while still retaining a strong predictive relationship.

As shown previously, the measure of consumption used in the estimation of PDI for an individual is the yearly consumption in kg of each of the 6 species. This translates into a relationship between estimated PDI and the "total yearly consumption" summed over all 6 species. Although the relationship between PDI and total yearly consumption is affected by the relative consumption of individual species, meal size and number of meals consumed, it was decided that this would be the best choice for the starting point of our simplified model, given that the aim was to relate estimated mercury intake (PDI) with consumption behaviour (total yearly consumption). A regression through the origin, of PDI on yearly total (see Figure 1), was run to find the cutoff point between predicted hazardous and non-hazardous consumption levels, for the sample population as a whole.

$$\mathrm{P\hat{D}I}_i = \hat{\beta} * total_i \qquad i = 1, \ldots, 880$$

where

$\hat{PDI}_i$ = the estimated daily intake for person *i*

$total_i$ = the total yearly consumption for person *i*

$\hat{\beta}$ = the estimated regression coefficient

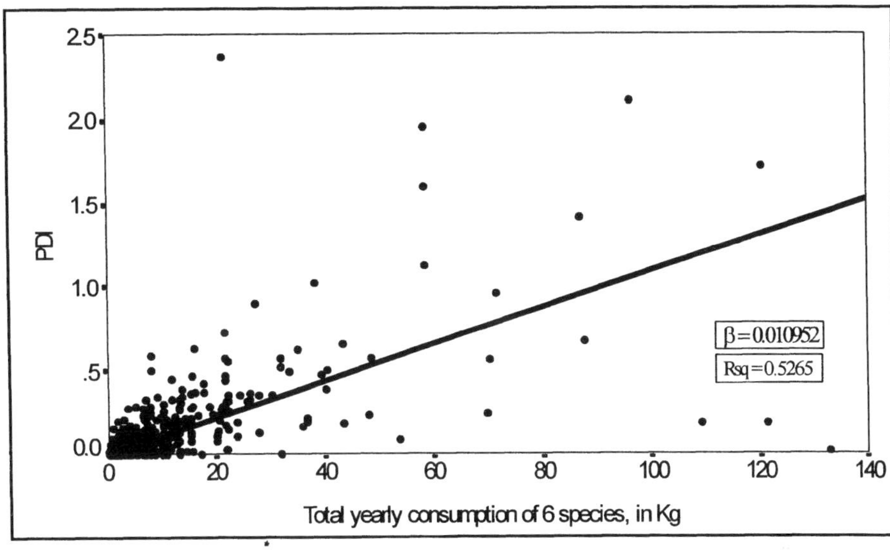

Figure 1 Relationship between estimated personal mercury intake and total fish consumption

Knowing the point at which PDI reaches a dangerous level (TDI of 0.47 μg/kgbw/day), it was then straightforward to calculate the maximum safe yearly consumption as

$$\text{max. safe } total = (\text{max. safe PDI}) / \hat{\beta}$$

This quantity was then translated into a monthly, rather than yearly, total as the time frame of interest. A lower limit was also placed on the total by replacing the estimated regression coefficient in the formula for the maximum safe total above, with the estimated coefficient plus 2 standard errors. As noted above, total consumption is a simple function of (meal size)×(number of meals). With the safe totals found above, this relation was used to calculate safe meal sizes for varying numbers of meals per month. This final version of the model for safe consumption levels would allow the user to choose either his/her meal size or number of meals, and alter the other quantity accordingly.

3. Results

The following results present information used from the two data files to execute the model. The first results section gives the EPS results, the second looks at the mercury levels in the fish, and the last section shows the results of applying the model. All results refer to the final sample of 880 individuals. The distribution of the sample by age and gender is shown in Table II.

		GENDER			
		Male	**Female**	**"Missing"**	**TOTAL**
AGE in years	**≤ 15**	105	106	2	213 (24.20%)
	16 - 45	213	213	-	426 (48.41%)
	46 - 60	67	62	-	129 (14.66%)
	> 60	46	53	-	99 (11.25%)
	"Missing"	7	6	-	13 (1.48%)
	TOTAL	438 (49.77%)	440 (50.00%)	2 (0.23%)	**880** (100%) (100%)

Table II Distribution of n=880 respondents by age and gender

3.1 EATING PATTERNS SURVEY

The average number of species consumed by the respondents is 2, although some respondents consumed all 6 species. The average meal size is 259 grams (range 42 to 697 grams) with an average number of meals per year of 21 (range 1 to 288 meals). The average and range of the number of meals per year would not have changed if the outliers had not been removed. However, meal weight would have ranged from 42 to 3344 grams per meal with a mean of 323 grams. This supports the idea that the meal size is a strong determining factor in the estimation of mercury intake levels and is why we decided to identify outliers on the basis of meal size.

Table III shows the total amount of each species consumed for all respondents. Pickerel surpasses any other species at 2204 kg per year. It is followed in order by whitefish at 822 kg per year, northern pike 687 kg per year, lake trout 586 kg per year, bass 579 kg per year, and perch at 566 kg per year.

3.2 MERCURY LEVELS

There are two main factors to consider when estimating the amount of mercury ingested: 1) the average level of mercury in each species around each community, and 2) the proportion of mercury ingested per species, for each individual.

The results in Table III show that pickerel had the highest average level of mercury, although three other species also had high levels, relative to the Canadian guideline for the sale of commercial fish of 0.5 ppm for total mercury. These were northern pike, lake trout

SPECIES	CONSUMPTION		MERCURY	
	TOTAL CONSUMPTION in Kg/year	% of TOTAL CONSUMPTION	MEAN[a] (Range[b]) in μg/g	MEAN % of PDI
PICKEREL	2204.25	40.49	0.56 (0.01 - 3.00)	55.63
WHITEFISH	821.72	15.10	0.15 (0.01 - 0.74)	9.10
NORTHERN PIKE	686.71	12.62	0.46 (0.03 - 1.40)	6.11
LAKE TROUT	585.68	10.76	0.41 (0.01 - 3.00)	6.49
BASS	579.09	10.64	0.38 (0.01 - 2.50)	8.20
PERCH	565.93	10.40	0.18 (0.01 - 0.61)	14.32

[a]average over all communities for the estimated mean levels for "big" fish (found through regression)
[b]range of levels over all fish sizes, from raw data

Table III Consumption and Mercury Levels by Species

and bass. When considering the second factor, pickerel accounts for more than 50% of the total personal intake of mercury. This is not surprising considering that pickerel is the most consumed and most contaminated species.

3.3 APPLICATION OF THE MODEL

Before discussing the identification of individuals with a high relative hazard, it is essential to review the extent to which this model covers true consumption by the participants. Because a perfect match between the species consumed and the species sampled and analyzed around a community is not possible, some controls are needed. In fact, this verification looks at the proportion of the consumption of the 6 selected species covered by the estimate. First, for 67% of the respondents, 100% of their consumption is covered by the model. That is, those respondents did not consume any species, or from any location, for which data was not available. Second, the model accounts on average for 87% of any respondent's total fish consumption.

The ultimate goal in examining fish consumption and fish contamination lies in using the relationship between the two to identify individuals whose relative hazard is high. As mentioned previously, this identification is a function of the relationship between the PDI and the TDI. The relationship has been measured two ways: 1) by defining whose relative hazard is high because of their exposure, and 2) by determining when and how people's relative hazard becomes high. If PDI $>$ TDI the individual's consumption is considered to be hazardous, if PDI $\leq$ TDI their consumption is considered non-hazardous.

For the purpose of this article, hazardous behaviour has been derived from an allocation scenario of 100% of the methylmercury TDI, as discussed earlier. This results in a total of 27 individuals (or 3.1%) being identified as having hazardous consumption behaviour. In determining an individual's relative hazard, gender is not a statistically significant factor.

Similarly, the respondent's age and weight do not influence the hazard status. The most important influencing factors appear to be the meal size, the number of meals consumed and the level of mercury as previously anticipated.

Even though the identification of the population displaying hazardous behaviour is a useful and interesting finding, our objective is to propose a model to estimate whether or not an individual's fish consumption is likely to result in a high relative hazard of mercury ingestion. Using the previously presented method, a meal weight / monthly number of meals grid with a hazardous consumption limit curve has been produced. Figure 2 allows the "safe" maximum meal size to be determined, given the number of meals consumed per month, or vice versa. Two curves have been drawn; the top curve gives the hazard limit, while the bottom curve is the hazard curve minus 2 standard errors (as explained earlier). The bottom curve provides the lowest "safe" consumption limit.

Any combination of meal size and number of meals per month which intersects above the upper curve would be considered hazardous behaviour. Two reference lines have been drawn in Figure 2 to provide population average information on the number of meals per month and the meal size. The intersection of these two lines represents the average monthly consumption parameters for the overall population. It can be seen that the average population is significantly below the hazard limit curve.

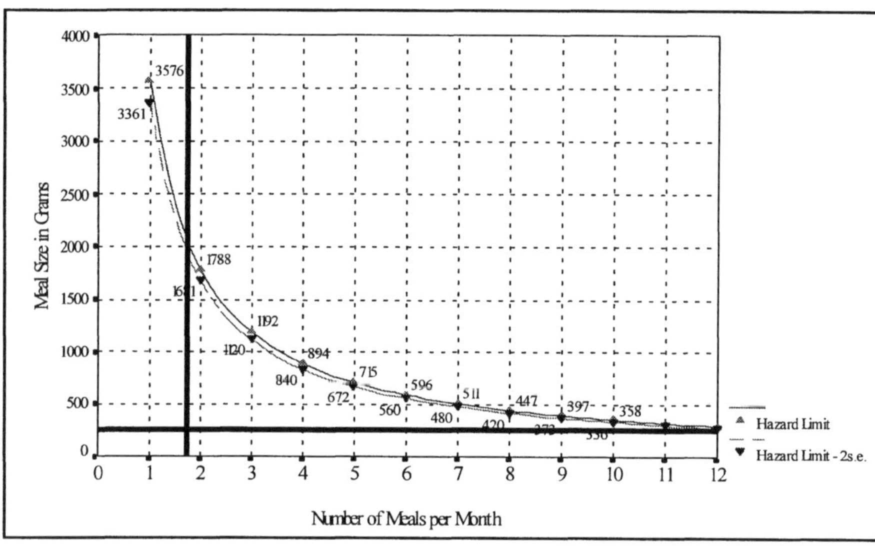

Figure 2. Fish Consumption Hazard Limit Curve for Great Lakes Basin First Nation Peoples

4. Discussion

Freshwater fish consumption remains one of the most significant indicators of continuing traditional lifestyle for First Nation Peoples of Canada. The development of a model for identifying individual hazardous behaviour can be used to promote "safer" consumption behaviour. The model substantiates the previously developed consumption guidelines and provides an uncomplicated way of establishing appropriate consumption patterns.

The results obtained through the process tend to confirm the usefulness of the model. With 67% of the respondents covered to 100% of consumption by the model, it can be agreed that this approach is positive for most people. However, in addition to usefulness, the issue of validity must also be addressed.

Although the standard error of the regression coefficient for the hazard limit is small (.00035034), it does not mean that the overall or cumulative error inherent in each step of the process has been taken into account. However, the model is sound using a statistical probabilistic error approach, although every level of error is not necessarily covered. This is what we wish to discuss in the next few lines.

Within the model development process, several different sources of error can be identified. The most important one is certainly the meal size. Because fish is consumed in different manners (fillet, soup, etc.) and because it has a varying density (thickness and volume of the fillet), the meal size is extremely difficult to estimate. Details on the estimation of meal size will be described in an EAGLE EPS report to be released in the coming year.

With regard to the mercury levels in the fish, some concerns and facts need to be recorded. The sampling program of MOEE surveys approximately 50 sites per year (not necessarily new sites) from which 10 to 20 samples per species are collected. If we consider the Ontario territory and its numerous lakes and rivers, we quickly conclude that it would be impossible to do an exhaustive and comprehensive sampling program in Canada.

The original samples tested by MOEE were collected by the Ministry of Natural Resources (MNR). Given that the MNR sampling is geared toward sport fishermen, the First Nation communities believe those sampling sites might not be the same locations as those where they go to fish . One component of the EAGLE Project was a fish sampling program, conducted during the years 1993-1995, to allow communities to collect samples from locations where they would usually go fishing, to provide more applicable data. It also collected samples for species largely consumed in the community, but previously undersampled.

Given the wide variety of species living in the Canadian lakes it is impossible to sample every one of them. Nevertheless, if we consider that, on average, 87% of the respondents' consumption is covered this shows adequate sampling.

Some analytical realities also have to be recognized. Contaminant analyses are extremely expensive and time consuming. Even if the sampling program was comprehensive, the laboratory work would be so significant that it would be impossible to keep up with the task.

Although TDIs represent established guidelines for determining "safe" consumption levels of individual contaminants, they are based on several assumptions that have been questioned in recent years including: *i*) The validity of extrapolating from effects in experimental animals to human populations; *ii*) The emphasis on acute effects on health, given that there is growing evidence that many contaminants can have chronic effects e.g., developmental effects, at doses lower than those that produce acute effects; *iii*) The use of highly variable safety factors; and *iv*) The validity of apportioning the TDI between different routes of exposure, i.e., water and food, and the validity of apportioning the assumed TDI for food between different types of food.

The model has been developed with the assumption that the average individual hazardous consumption pattern could be identified, although it does not take into account cases of point source contamination or extreme consumers. However, the model does include some factors that make it conservative in nature. First, the most consumed species (pickerel) also contains the highest levels of mercury. Second, the model assumes consumption of the "big" size fish which is larger and therefore results in a higher estimated mercury level than the average fish. Finally, the high relative hazard population has a much larger consumption level than the average population. For these reasons, we believe the model to have a considerable built-in safety factor.

There are still some concerns which will need to be addressed in the future to determine the level of quality and usefulness of the model. Field testing needs to be carried out to assess the strength of the model's predictive ability. One possibility for this is to obtain actual mercury levels in hair, from a subset of the sample population used to create the model. Practical application of the model is also likely to suggest possible improvements for future work.

Acknowledgements

The authors wish to thank the members of the EAGLE First Nations communities and the EAGLE Project without whose collaboration and coordination the development of the model would not have been possible. We would also like to thank the Ontario Ministry of Environment and Energy for their invaluable assistance and contribution to the project and recognize funding from the Health Canada Action Plan on Health and the Environment (Green Plan).

References

Birke, G., Johnels, A.G., Plantin, L., Sjöstrand, B., Skerfving, S., and Westermark,T.: 1972, Studies on Humans Exposed to Methyl Mercury Through Fish Consumption. *Archives of Environmental Health*, 25, 77-91.

EAGLE: 1996a, EAGLE Eating Patterns Survey Final Report. (in preparation).

EAGLE: 1996b, EAGLE Final Report on Risk Assessment from Fish Consumption. (in preparation).

Fleming, L.E., Watkins, S., Kaderman, R., Levin, B., Ayyar, D.R., Bizzo, M., Stephens, D., and Bean, J.A.: 1995, Mercury Exposure in Humans Through Food Consumption from the Everglades of Florida. *Water, Air, and Soil Pollution*, 80, 41-48.

Hovinga, M.E., Sowers, M., and Humphrey, H.E.B.: 1993, Environmental Exposure and Lifestyle Predictors of Lead, Cadmium, PCB, and DDT Levels in Great Lakes Fish Eaters. *Archives of Environmental Health*, 48, 98-104.

Kyle, J.H., and Ghani, N.: 1982, Methylmercury in Human Hair: A Study of a Papua New Guinean Population Exposed to Methylmercury through Fish Consumption. *Archives of Environmental Health*, 37, 266-270.

MOEE: 1995, *1995-1996 Guide to Eating Ontario Sport Fish*. Ontario Ministry of Environment and Energy, Toronto.

Richardson, M., Egyed, M., and Currie, D. J.: 1995, Human Exposure To Mercury May Decrease As Acidic Deposition Increases. *Water, Air, and Soil Pollution*, 80, 31-39.

Ricker, W. E.: 1979, Growth Rates and Models, in *Fish Physiology, Vol VIII Bioenergetics and Growth*. Hoar, W. S., Randall, D. J., and Brett, J. R. eds. 677-743.

WHO: 1990, *Environmental Health Criteria 101, Methylmercury*. International Programme on Chemical Safety, Geneva.

Wheatley, B. and Paradis, S.: 1995, Exposure of Canadian Aboriginal Peoples to Methylmercury. *Water, Air, and Soil Pollution*, 80, 3-11.

Wheatley, B. and Paradis, S.: 1996, Balancing Human Exposure, Risk and Reality: Questions Raised by the Canadian Aboriginal Methylmercury Program. *NeuroToxicology*, 17(1), 241-250.

PROBABILISTIC ASSESSMENT OF REGIONAL MERCURY EXPOSURE

C. SEIGNEUR[1], P. PAI[1], M. GERATH[2,3], D. MITCHELL[2], G. HAMBY[2], G. GONG[2], C. WHIPPLE[4], AND L. LEVIN[5]

[1]AER, 2682 Bishop Drive, Suite 120, San Ramon, California 94583.
[2]ENSR, 35 Nagog Park, Acton, Massachusetts 01720.
[2]Current address: Ogden, 239 Littleton Road, Suite 7C, Westford, Massachusetts 01886.
[4]ICF Kaiser, 1800 Harrison Street, Oakland, California 94612.
[5]Electric Power Research Institute, 3412 Hillview Avenue, Palo Alto, California 94303.

Abstract. A methodology for the probabilistic assessment of regional exposure to mercury is presented. The methodology is based on a multimedia model of the atmospheric fate and transport of mercury over a continental scale, and the aquatic simulation of the transformation and bioaccumulation of mercury in lakes in the region of interest. A probabilistic approach allows one to take into account the spatial variability of environmental characteristics and the variability of dose-related variables (e.g., fish consumption, body weight) among individuals. The methodology is demonstrated for total mercury deposition in the Great Lakes region of the U.S.

1. Introduction

Previous work has focused on the health risk assessment of mercury (Hg) emissions from industrial facilities such as power plants at local spatial scales, i.e., of the order of 100 km (e.g., Constantinou *et al.*, 1995a). Since recent studies have shown that the local impacts (i.e., within 100 km) of Hg emissions from individual power plants are typically not significant and that the majority of these power plant emissions is transported beyond 100 km from the sources (Allan *et al.*, 1994; Constantinou *et al.*, 1995b), it is of interest to address the potential impacts of Hg emissions at regional scales (i.e., at scales ranging from 100 km to several 1,000 km). We address here the potential regional impacts of atmospheric Hg transported over the contiguous United States of America (U.S.). Figure 1 depicts the overall methodology used to assess the potential exposure to Hg transported over such regional scales. This methodology consists of the following steps:

(1) Simulation of the long-range transport, transformations and deposition of atmospheric Hg over a continental scale;
(2) Simulation of the aquatic chemistry and bioaccumulation in fish of Hg in lakes of a selected region;
(3) Estimation of the human dose of Hg through consumption of local freshwater fish.

Clearly, it is not feasible to simulate the fate and bioaccumulation of Hg in fish for every surface water body of the contiguous U.S. Moreover, consumption of fish from local lakes varies significantly among individuals. Therefore, a probabilistic approach was selected that could account for the spatial variability of environmental characteristics relevant to the atmospheric deposition and bioaccumulation of Hg, as well as for the variability in local fish consumption among the U.S. population. In this

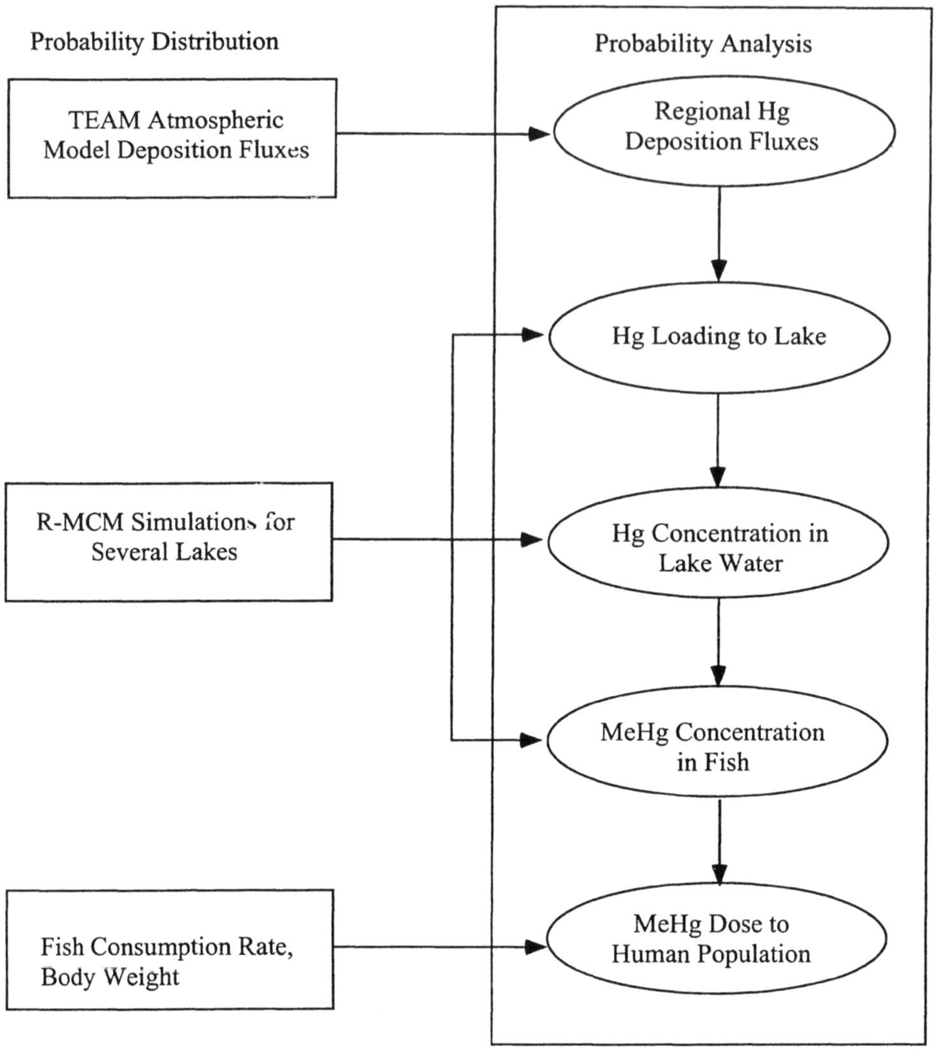

Fig. 1. Schematic Description of the Methodology for the Probabilistic Assessment of Regional Hg Exposure.

approach, we use probability distributions of the major relevant variables to construct probability distributions of the human exposure to Hg through fish consumption. It must be emphasized that there are large uncertainties that remain in various components of the analysis (i.e., atmospheric modeling, aquatic modeling, dose modeling). Our analysis addresses only the variability of key input variables and does not include a treatment of input data uncertainties or model formulation uncertainties. Therefore, the results presented here should be seen as a demonstration of the methodology rather than definitive exposure assessment values. It must be noted also that our regional assessment addresses all sources of Hg, not only power plant emissions. Global background Hg is included through the boundary conditions of the atmospheric model. However, since our analysis addresses the regional impacts of Hg emissions, the localized impacts of specific sources (air emissions, water discharges or land contamination) are not considered. Also, it should be noted that at this point, uncertainties still remain in emission speciation, boundary conditions, meteorological inputs and model formulation that prevent us from using the models for the purpose of estimating individual contributions from specific sources.

We present first the overall modeling approach. Next, the probability distributions selected for the relevant variables are discussed. Then, the methodology is demonstrated using the Great Lakes region of the U.S. as an example.

2. Modeling Approach

As depicted in Figure 1, the overall model of the fate and transport of Hg and its dose to humans consists of several components. We briefly discuss each of these components.

Atmospheric transport, transformation and deposition of Hg: The TEAM regional atmospheric model (Pai *et al.*, 1997) was used to simulate the long-range transport, chemical transformations, and dry and wet deposition of Hg over the contiguous U.S. Comparison of the simulation results of the TEAM model with observations for total gaseous Hg (TGM) ambient concentrations and wet deposition fluxes showed reasonable agreement (Pai *et al.*, 1997). Therefore, the dry and wet deposition fluxes of Hg calculated by the TEAM atmospheric model were used as input to the watersheds.

Hg loading to the lake: The amount of Hg that enters a lake depends on the total Hg loading to the watershed from atmospheric deposition (see above), the ratio of the watershed area to the lake area and the fraction of Hg deposited in the watershed that is transported to the lake. The Regional Mercury Cycling Model (R-MCM) (Harris *et al.*, 1996) was used to simulate Hg loading to lakes from dry and wet deposition fluxes to their watersheds.

Hg methylation in lake water and bioaccumulation in fish: The aquatic concentration of methylHg and its bioaccumulation through the food chain depend on the Hg loading to the lake, the characteristics of the lake (water quality, acidity, watershed type, biological characteristics) and the bioenergetics of the various trophic levels from bentos to predator fishes. R-MCM was used to simulate the cycling of Hg in lakes and its bioaccumulation in fish.

Ingestion dose: The methylHg dose to the human body depends on the methylHg concentration in fish, the consumption rate of fish caught in local lakes and the human body weight. Note that we consider only methylHg as the Hg species of interest. Also, we only address here the consumption of local freshwater fish. Consumption of commercial fish from freshwater and the ocean/sea will contribute to the total body burden, but their methylHg concentrations are not addressed in our modeling approach, since some of those fishes reside out of our modeling domain. Consumption of commercial fish can be considered to be a "background" fish intake and we address here the incremental fish intake due to consumption of fish caught by local anglers.

The mathematical relationships for each one of these model components are presented below. Note that in each case, a relatively sophisticated model (e.g., TEAM, R-MCM) is used to develop a range of parameter values (e.g., atmospheric deposition flux, bioaccumulation factor) for input into the probabilistic model.

The atmospheric deposition flux (ADF) (μg/(m^2•y)) is calculated as the sum of the dry deposition flux, DDF, and wet deposition flux, WDF, obtained from the TEAM atmospheric model.

$$ADF = DDF + WDF \quad (1)$$

The Hg loading to lakes, MLL (μg/(m^2•y)) is calculated by R-MCM for each given lake.

$$MLL = ADF * W \quad (2)$$

where W is a dimensionless parameter that is lake-specific. This parameter accounts for the ratio of the watershed area to the lake area, as well as the fraction of Hg retained in the terrestrial area surrounding the lake.

The total Hg concentration in the lake water column, C_w (mg/l) depends on the Hg loading to the lake as well as some lake-specific characteristics such as the sedimentation rate.

$$C_w = MLL * d * 10^{-6} \quad (3)$$

where d is a lake-specific parameter (y/m) that is calculated by R-MCM.

The methylation of Hg in lake water and its bioaccumulation in fish were found to be slightly negatively correlated in the application of R-MCM to 29 lakes throughout the U.S. That is, there were no lakes with both high methylation rate and high bioaccumulation factors. Therefore, the processes of Hg methylation and subsequent bioaccumulation were grouped into a single equation that represents the ratio of methylHg concentration in fish, C_f (mg/kg) to total Hg concentration in lake water, C_w.

$$C_f = C_w * BAF_t \quad (4)$$

where BAF_t represents a bioaccumulation factor referring to total Hg in lake water (l/kg). BAF_t is a lake-specific parameter that is calculated by R-MCM.

The ingestion dose rate, D (mg/(kg•day)), is calculated from the methylHg fresh fish concentration, C_f, the fish consumption rate, FIR (g/day) and the human body weight, BW (kg).

$$D = C_f * FIR * 10^{-3} / BW \quad (5)$$

3. Probability Distributions of Input Variables and Parameters

For the purpose of demonstrating the methodology, we apply it to the Great Lakes region. We present here the probability distributions selected for the relevant variables for this specific application. As mentioned above, the TEAM atmospheric model was used to estimate the deposition fluxes of Equation (1), and R-MCM was used to calculate the parameters W, d, and BAF_t in Equations (2) through (4).

The atmospheric model, TEAM, was applied to an area that covers the contiguous U.S., southern Canada and northern Mexico. Hg deposition fluxes due to the global background and anthropogenic Hg emissions from within the TEAM domain were simulated over the entire domain. Results are presented here for the Great Lakes region. A comparison of TEAM model simulation results for atmospheric TGM concentrations and Hg wet deposition fluxes with observations collected in Minnesota, Wisconsin and Michigan showed the model calculations to be consistent with the observations (Pai *et al.*, 1997). For the purpose of this probabilistic assessment, we selected the full range of modeled deposition values for three states of the Great Lakes area (Minnesota, Wisconsin and Michigan) to represent the variable DDF and WDF of Equation (1). These three states correspond to states where lakes simulated with R-MCM were located. Values of the deposition fluxes were calculated by the atmospheric model for each surface grid cell of 100 km x 100 km area. Lognormal distributions represented most closely the deposition flux histograms and, therefore, were selected for both dry and wet deposition fluxes. The characteristics of these distributions are presented in Table I.

Table I.
Input Variables used in the Probabilistic Exposure Assessment.

Input Variable	Distribution Function	Characteristics	Source
DDF	Lognormal truncated[1,3]	Mean = 5.1 μg/(m^2•y) σ = 2.8 μg/(m^2•y)	TEAM
WDF	Lognormal truncated[1,3]	Mean = 8.4 μg/(m^2•y) σ = 4.6 μg/(m^2•y)	TEAM
W	Lognormal truncated[2,3]	Mean = 2.42 σ = 0.38	R-MCM
d	Lognormal truncated[2,3]	Mean = 45.4 y/m σ = 26.3 y/m	R-MCM
BAF_t	Lognormal truncated[2,3]	Mean = 390,000 l/kg σ = 218,000 l/kg	R-MCM
FIR	0 up to 65th percentile, Exponential truncated above 65th percentile	Mean = 3.7 g/day Maximum value = 200 g/day	This work
BW	Lognormal[3]	Mean = 66 kg σ = 13 kg	AIHC, 1994

[(1)]Distributions were truncated at the minimum and maximum values obtained in the TEAM simulation.
[(2)]Distributions were truncated at two standard deviations above the mean or at the maximum value obtained in the 8 R-MCM simulations, whichever was the greater.
[(3)]Arithmetic mean and standard deviation.

R-MCM was applied to a data base of 29 lakes distributed throughout the U.S. (Mitchell *et al.*, 1995) with 8 of those lakes located in the Great Lakes region, in Minnesota, Wisconsin and Michigan. These eight lakes include drainage lakes as well as seepage lakes. Table II summarizes the major characteristics of these eight lakes.

Table II
Summary of Lake Characteristics

Lake number & name	Lake Type	pH	DOC (mg/l)	Predatory Fish Species
1. McGrath L.	Seepage	5.4	3.0	Largemouth bass
2. L. Mendota	Drainage	8.5	10.0	Walleye
3. Big Portage L.	Drainage	8.6	3.0	Northern pike
4. L. Mitchell	Drainage	7.7	3.0	Walleye
5. Park L.	Seep./Drain.	8.3	12.6	Largemouth bass
6. Platte L.	Drainage	8.3	2.0	Northern pike
7. Grove L.	Drainage	8.1	10.0	Northern pike
8. Mountain L.	Drainage	7.4	10.0	Northern pike

The median, mean and maximum values for methylHg concentration in predator fish for the eight lakes simulated are 0.46, 0.67 and 2.1 ppm, respectively. These results are commensurate with observed methylHg concentrations in fish observed in the Great Lakes region. For example, a survey of 56 lakes in Michigan gave an arithmetic mean concentration of methylHg in largemouth bass (all ages) of 0.44 ppm and a maximum concentration of 1.8 ppm (Day, 1996). Figure 2 presents the modeled methylated fraction of Hg for these lakes; Figure 3 presents the modeled bioaccumulation factor for methylHg (the product of these two parameters correspond to BAF_t in Equation (4)). The methylHg concentrations in fish were found to be sensitive primarily to the dissolved organic carbon concentration in lake water, lake temperature, pH and sediment burial velocity. The results of the R-MCM simulations showed significant variation in methylHg concentrations and methylHg bioaccumulation in fish, within a given region (e.g., in the Great Lakes region as shown in Figures 2 and 3). These variations result from the differences in water quality that can be observed among surface water bodies within a given region. Therefore, it would not be feasible to represent a region by a single "typical" lake, and a probabilistic approach that integrates the variations in environmental characteristics observed within that region is the preferred approach. The R-MCM simulation results for these eight lakes were used to develop probability distributions of the parameters W, d, and BAF_t. The application of R-MCM to the data base of 29 lakes suggests that the variability of these parameters can be approximated by lognormal distributions. The specific distributions derived for the Great Lakes region are presented in Table I.

The probability distribution for the fish consumption rate was developed as follows. The mean consumption in the U.S. population, including those who eat freshwater fish and those who do not, is estimated to be 2.2 g/day based on the 1989-1991 Continuous Survey of Food Intake by Individuals (CSFII) conducted by the U.S. Department of the Agriculture (EPA, 1996). This freshwater fish consumption includes both locally caught fish and farm raised fish. The latter amounts to a production of over 500 million pounds per year, i.e., about 2.4 g/day per capita. However, only about half of this amount is likely to be eaten due to wastage and the fact that not all of the production weight is edible. This analysis suggests that the average consumption of locally caught

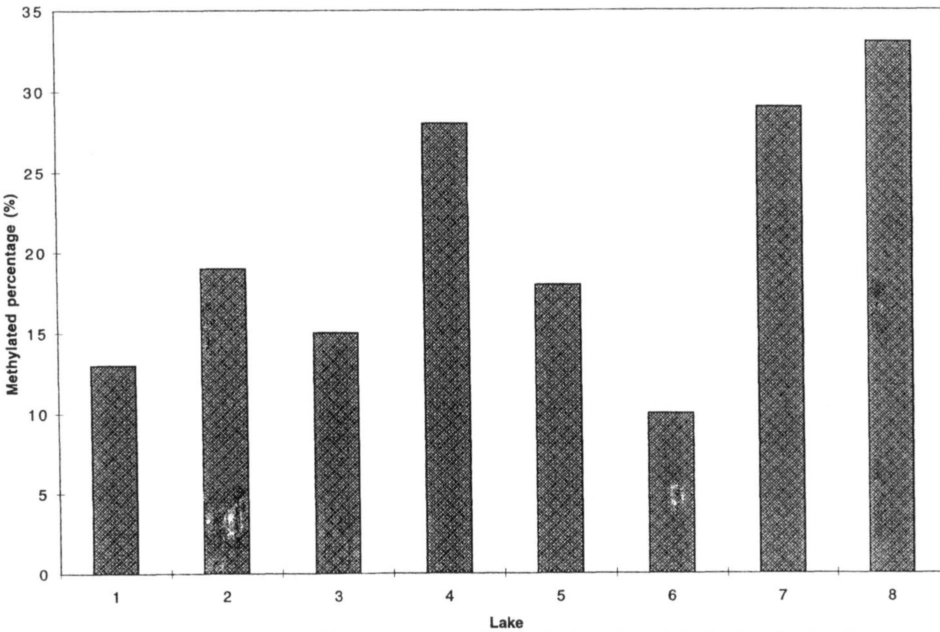

Fig. 2. Calculated Methylated Percentage of Hg in Lakes for eight Lakes in the Great Lakes Region.

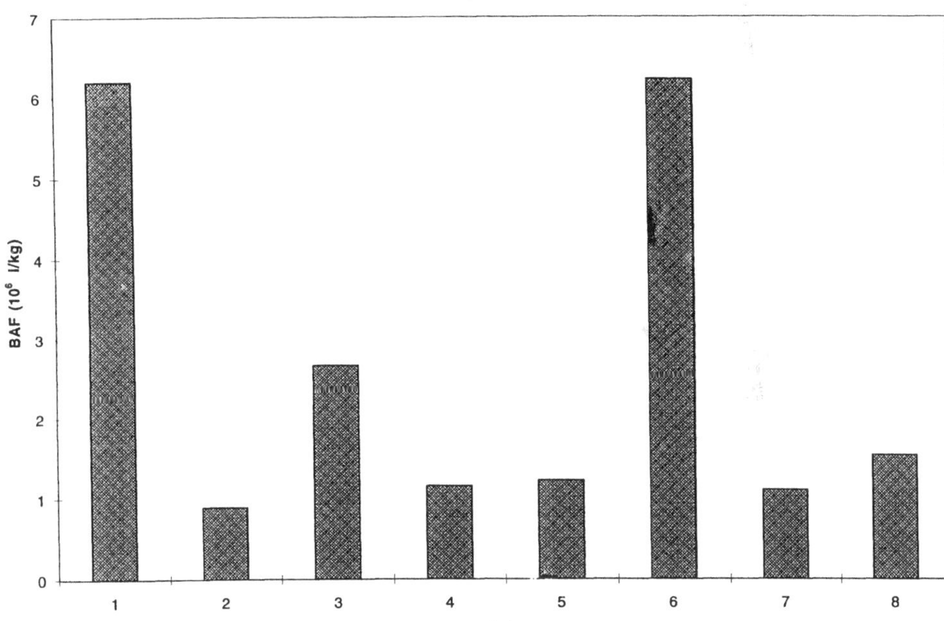

Fig. 3. MethylHg Bioaccumulation Factor calculated for the Predator Fish for eight Lakes in the Great Lakes Region.

fish is of the order of 1 g/day. The U. S. Environmental Protection Agency (EPA) Mercury Study Report to Congress cites a U.S. Fish and Wildlife Service report indicating that 26% of the U.S. population fished in 1985 (EPA, 1996). The EPA report also provides a review of fish consumption among groups of anglers. Ten studies are reported in the EPA report. There is a large variation in the amount of locally caught fish consumed by the anglers. The mean (or, if not available, the median) value reported in these studies ranges from 1.8 g/day (Soldat, 1970) to 60 g/day (Sekerke *et al.*, 1994). Ebert *et al.* (1993) reported in a study of Maine anglers a mean value of 5.0 g/day for fish consumption by all surveyed anglers and 3.7 g/day for fish consumption by the anglers and their family. Combining the results reported by Ebert *et al.* and the EPA estimate that 26% of the population fishes recreationally suggests that 35% of the population eats locally caught freshwater fish. These values result in a mean consumption rate of 1.3 g/day for the entire U.S. population, which is consistent with the estimate based on the CSFII data base. Based on this review of available data, we assumed that 65% of the population does not eat locally caught freshwater fish. For the 35% of the population that does consume locally caught freshwater fish, an exponential distribution with a mean value of 3.7 g/day and truncated at a maximum value of 200 g/day was used. An exponential type distribution is consistent with the review of freshwater fish consumption assessments.

The probability distribution for the weight of an adult woman is based on the work of Brainard and Burmaster (1992) and is recommended in the American Industrial Health Council's Exposure Factors Sourcebook (AIHC, 1994). The distribution is lognormal with an arithmetic mean value of 66 kg. A correlation between the fish consumption rate and the body weight was introduced to account for the fact that heavier individuals tend to eat more. A value of 0.33 was used for the correlation coefficient, following Hoover *et al.* (1997), who derived their correlation based on data reported in Lipfert *et al.* (1996).

4. Probabilistic Exposure Assessment

The model presented in Section 2 was applied in a probabilistic mode to the Great Lakes region using the probability distributions presented in Section 3. The Crystal Ball software (Decisioneering, 1992) was used to conduct a Monte Carlo simulation with 15,000 iterations. (The sensitivity of the probabilistic assessment was tested by comparing the results obtained with 15,000 and 20,000 iterations; no significant changes were observed between the two simulations.)

The results for methylHg concentrations in predator fish (i.e., largemouth bass, walleye or northern pike) are presented in Figure 4. The mean value is 0.46 ppm and the maximum value is 4.4 ppm. The 50th (median), 60th, 70th, 80th and 90th percentiles of the distribution are 0.36, 0.44, 0.54, 0.68 and 0.92 ppm, respectively. These results are commensurate with the observed methylHg concentrations in fish in Michigan lakes that were mentioned above. The maximum value modeled in the probabilistic analysis is greater than the maximum value obtained in lake-specific simulations because the former combines atmospheric deposition, hydrology and water quality variables conducive to high Hg fish concentrations. The results for the human dose simulation are presented in Figure 5. The distribution shows a median value of zero since it is assumed that 65% of the population does not eat fish caught in local water bodies. Therefore, according to our analysis, their incremental dose is zero. The mean value of the modeled dose is 8.9×10^{-6}

mg/(kg•day). The 70th, 80th and 90th percentiles of the distribution are 2.4×10^{-6}, 1.0×10^{-5} and 2.6×10^{-5} mg/(kg•day), respectively; the maximum value is 5.7×10^{-4} mg/(kg•day). It must be noted that uncertainties remain in the various steps of this exposure assessment model and that the results presented here must be seen as exploratory and primarily as a demonstration of a methodology of the regional assessment of Hg potential exposure.

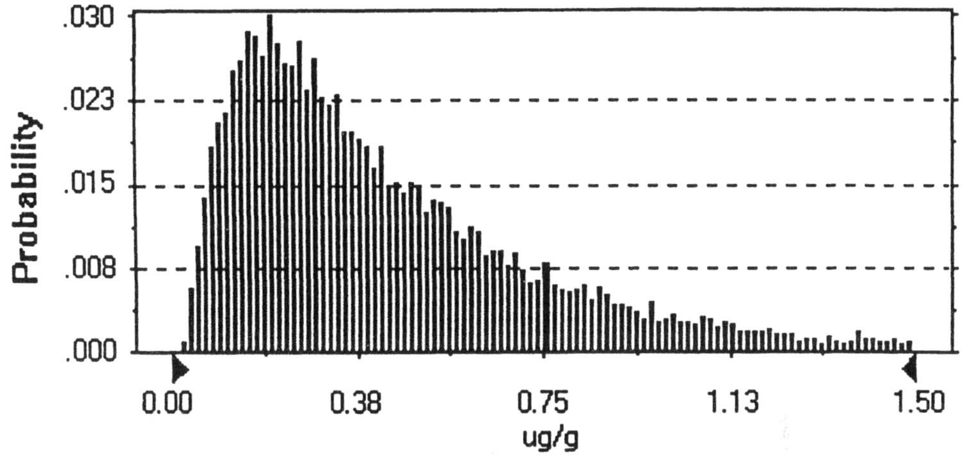

Fig. 4. Probability Distribution of the Modeled MethylHg Concentration in Fish.

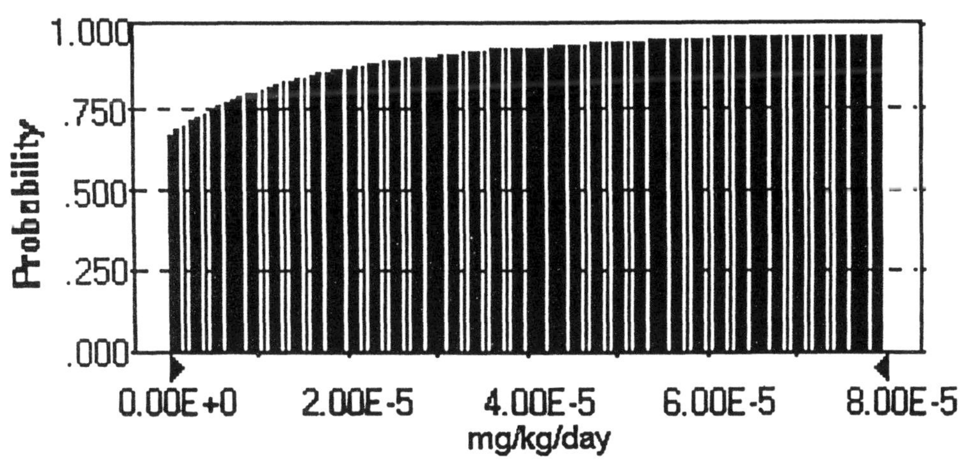

Fig. 5. Cumulative Distribution of the Modeled Human Dose due to Local Fish Consumption

5. Summary

A methodology for the health risk assessment of Hg at regional scales has been presented. The methodology combines atmospheric modeling at a continental scale, modeling of Hg cycling and bioaccumulation in lakes of a region within the continental domain, and modeling of Hg intake by the local population through fish consumption. Because of the spatial variability of many environmental characteristics and variability of exposure parameters among individuals, a probabilistic approach was selected. The methodology was demonstrated through its application to the Great Lakes region. Further work will focus on the following items: (1) The methodology will be extended to include uncertainties in the model input data in addition to the variability in the parameters, (2) the regional exposure assessment will be extended to other regions (e.g., the northeastern U.S. and Florida) where lake contamination by atmospheric Hg is of concern, and, (3) to the extent possible, R-MCM simulations of Hg concentrations in fish will be compared to available data for specific lakes in various regions of the U.S.

Acknowledgements

This work was funded under projects WO-3508-02 and WO-3508-03 from the Electric Power Research Institute (EPRI), Palo Alto, California. Thanks are due to Ms. K. Lohman, AER, Ms. K. Wandland, ENSR, and Ms. B. Ruffle, ENSR, for their assistance with the data and computations, and Ms. E. Constantinou, for her comments. We are also grateful to Dr. R. Harris, TetraTech, Inc.; Dr. D. Porcella, EPRI and Mr. N. Bloom, Frontier Geosciences, Inc., for useful discussions during the course of this study.

References

AIHC: 1994, *Exposure Factors Sourcebook*, American Industrial Health Council, Washington, D.C.

Allan, M. A., Levin, L., Porcella, D., Silvers, A., Wyzga, R., Chang, R., Chu, P., Nott, B., Owens, D. and Toole-O'Neil, B.: 1994, *Electric Utility Trace Substances Synthesis Report, Vol. 3, Appendix O, Mercury in the Environment*, TR-104614-V3, Electric Power Research Institute, Palo Alto, California.

Brainard, J. and Burmaster, D.: 1992, *Risk Analysis*, **12**, 267-275.

Constantinou, E., Gerath, M., Mitchell, D., Seigneur, C. and Levin, L.: 1995a, *Water Air Soil Pollut.*, **80**, 1129-1138.

Constantinou, E., Wu, X. A. and Seigneur, C.: 1995b, *Water Air Soil Pollut.*, **80**, 325-335.

Day, R.: 1996, Electronic data base, Michigan Department of Environmental Quality, Lansing, Michigan.

Decisioneering, Inc.: 1996, *Crystal Ball for Windows*, User's Manual.

Ebert, E. S., Harrington, N. W., Boyle, K. J., Knight, J. W. and Keenan, R. E.: 1993, *North American J. Fisheries Manag.*, **13**, 737-745.

EPA: 1995, *Exposure Factors Handbook*, draft, U.S. Environmental Protection Agency, Washington, D.C.

EPA: 1996, *Mercury Study Report to Congress, Appendix H*, EPA-452/R-96-001, U.S. Environmental Protection Agency, Washington, D.C.

Harris, R., Gherini, S. and Hudson, R.: 1996, *Regional Mercury Cycling Model: A Model for Mercury Cycling in Lakes, R-MCM Version 1.0, Draft User Guide and Technical Reference*, prepared for the Electric Power Research Institute and the Wisconsin Department of Natural Resources, TetraTech, Inc., Lafayette, California.

Hoover, S., Hill, R. and Watson, T.: 1997, *Water Air Soil Pollut.*, in press.

Lipfert, F. W., Moskowitz, P. D., Fthenakis, V. and Saroff, L.: 1996, *Neurotox.*, **17**, 197-212.

Mitchell, D., Mounce, T., Hamby, G., Chia, G., Abeck, H., Vertucci, F. and Seigneur, C.: 1995, *Regional Limnological Database for Mercury Cycling Modeling*, Report No. 2460-025-700 to the Electric Power Research Institute, ENSR, Acton, Massachusetts.

Pai, P., Karamchandani, P. and Seigneur, C.: 1997, *Atmos. Environ.*, in press.

Sekerke, H. J., Denger, R. L., Adams, C. M. and Moss, S. D.: 1994, Abstract No. 563, Society of Toxicology 33rd Annual Meeting.

Soldat, J. K.: 1970, in *Environmental Surveillance in the Vicinity of Nuclear Facilities*, Rienig, W. C., ed., Thomas, Springfield, Illinois, 302-308.

THE HEALTH SAFETY PROGRAMME FOR WORKERS EXPOSED TO ELEMENTAL MERCURY AT THE MERCURY MINE IN IDRIJA

A. KOBAL , T. DIZDAREVIČ

Idrija Mercury Mine, Arkova 43, 5280 Idrija, Slovenia

Abstract. In the Idrija Mine ore appears in two forms: the first as cinnabar (70%) and the second as native mercury (30%). In the area where native mercury was mined the concentrations of elemental mercury in the working and unventilated areas of the pit were very high, they periodically reached over and above 3 mg/m^3 of air and most of the time exceeded the maximum acceptable levels of mercury vapours in the air (0.1 mg/m^3). In such specific working conditions the number of workers suffering from the effects of mercury was very high. Work conditions in the mine urgently required more effective and preventative measures against exposure to mercury. The health and safety program includes monitoring of mercury concentrations, technical measures, personal protection, evaluation of individual external intensity of exposure and medical surveillance. The results were very successful; the number of mercury intoxicated workers dropped and after 1975 there were no more intoxicated workers, in spite of the increase in the number of areas worked where native mercury was present.

1. Introduction

In its 500-year history (1490-1994), the Idrija Mine has produced a total of 147,000 tons of commercial mercury, which represents over 13% of the entire world production to date. The Idrija deposit is situated below the centre of the town of Idrija. It is 1500 m long (the width of the orebody deposits ranges from 300 m to 600 m) and 450 m deep. Ore appears in two forms: 70% as cinnabar (HgS), and 30% as native mercury (Hg) Cinnabar is the main ore mineral. In the entire ore-containing zone there are more than 140 orebodies of cinnabar and 15 orebodies composed of native mercury in permocarboniferous schist. The Idrija Mine has its own ore deposits from which the mercury ore was extracted, and a smeltery in which elemental mercury was produced. The operation of both plants was closely connected, both technically and economically.

Until 1975, the Idrija Mine mainly exploited orebodies of variable cinnabar content. In addition to cinnabar ore, smaller amounts of elemental mercury also appeared regularly in rich orebodies. During the entire 500 years of the Mine's operation, miners therefore tended to avoid the excavation of carboniferous schist and preferred to excavate cinnabar ore around the schist in solid rock. However, due to the low mercury content of the cinnabar orebodies, the increasing need appeared for mining orebodies in carboniferous schist (after 1975) in which the mercury appears in a predominantly elemental form (Hg^0). The technology of the processing of mercury ore changed and was improved over the years after the second world war by the replacement of shaft furnaces and Špirek furnaces, with today's rotary furnaces.

The production of mercury and at the same time also the number of employees reached their peaks in the 18th century and in the period after the second world war until 1977 (Table I). Mercury production was temporarily stopped from 1978 to 1982, and resumed in 1983 until 1994, when the final shutdown of the Mine began.

Table I. The number of employees and extracted amounts of mercury (Mohori~ 1960, Archive of Safety Dept.).

Period	Number of employees	Extracted quantities of Hg (tons/year)
16th century	100 - 200	30
17th century	350	50 - 250
18th century	600 - 1350	250 - 700
19th century	600	270
20th century (until 1977)	800 - 1100	500
1983 - 1992	200	45
1995	140	0

From the very beginnings of the extraction and processing of ore in the Mine, miners and smelters were exposed to the harmful effects of mercury during their work. The number of intoxications with mercury among miners and smelters was exceptionally high in the first twenty years following the Second World War due to extremely high concentrations of mercury in the working environment.

In view of the mentioned facts, it was evident at the time that the main problem concerning the protection of workers was how to prevent or reduce the number of occupational intoxications with mercury. In our contribution we have presented the main health and safety problems of mercury exposed workers and the basic concepts and orientations of the Health Safety Programme aimed at protecting the work abilities of workers exposed to elemental mercury (Hg^0).

2. Materials and methods

In the first part of our contribution we evaluated the incidence of mercury intoxications, the work conditions and exposure to Hg^0 after the second world war. The second part of our contribution presents the basic concept and the application of the Health Safety Programme, which was introduced after 1965 in the Idrija Mercury Mine. This programme was based on large research activities particularly in the field of technical protective measures, monitoring of mercury concentrations in the work places, evaluation of individual intensity of exposure, biological monitoring and target medical examinations.

Our contribution is focused primarily on presenting the development of methodological changes in the fields of safety and health of workers exposed to Hg^0. More significant methods and techniques used shall be indicated in individual subchapters of our contribution by references to their authors. Only the methodology of medical examinations and methods of analysis shall be presented separately.

TARGET MEDICAL EXAMINATION

The medical surveillance of workers exposed to elevated mercury concentrations (above 0.1 mg/m^3 of air) was performed by means of target medical examinations and biological monitoring (Zielhuis 1978). We based the target medical examinations on the experiences of different authors (Trachtenberg 1972, WHO 1976) and our own experiences (Kobal 1975a, 1991). Specific questions were asked regarding typical nonspecific neuropsychical symptoms (sleep disturbances, anxiety, depression, fatigue, decreasing memory, paraesthesia, cramps in leg muscles, tremor and irritability), oral and gastrointestinal symptoms. Clinical examination was performed at the level of medical screening. The examination also included neurological status with a subjective classification, including postural tremor of the upper extremity, coordination, reflexes, the presence or absence of pathological reflex including snout reflex and pin-pain sensation, touch pressure, two-point discrimination and vibratory sensation (using a 128 Hz tuning fork). Quantitative examination of clinical and subclinal signs was not included.

ANALYTICAL METHODS

Hg^0 in the air was determined by UV photometry using two portable instruments. These were a Beckmann mercury vapour meter (K-23) and a mercury vapour indicator (MVI) designed to detect minute concentrations. The K-23 was calibrated in mg/m^3 in the range from 0.005 to 0.1 and 0.003 to 3.0, reproducibility $\pm$ 10%. The MVI is calibrated in $\mu g/m^3$ in the range from 0.0 to 2000.0, with a sensitivity of 1 $\mu g/m^3$, reproducibility $\pm$ 5%.

Stationary sampling of pit air was also made by the aspiration of air through a $KMnO_4$ solution by means of battery-operated pumps at a flow rate of 1-2 l/min. The sampling time varied from 15 to 90 minutes. The samples were analyzed by means of the dithizon method until 1970 and later by a cold vapour atomic absorption technique (MAS Perkin Elmer apparatus, Model 50, Coleman) (Hatch and Ott 1968). After 1986 the mercury concentrations in the samples of $KMnO_4$ solution were analyzed by cold vapour atomic absorption spectrometrie (CVAAS) (Horvat 1989).

Before 1970 the urine mercury was analyzed by the dithizone method, later by the above mentioned vapour atomic absorption technique. In 1986 urine mercury and also blood mercury was determined by reduction - amalgamation cold vapour atomic absorption spectrometrie

(Horvat 1989). The limit of urine mercury (U-Hg) detection was 0.1 ng/g in a 0.5g sample with a variability coefficient (depending on the concentration) of 5 - 10 %. The mercury concentrations in urine spot samples were usually corrected for a specific gravity of 1024 (Barber, Wallis 1986).

3. Results and Discussion

INCIDENCE OF MERCURY INTOXICATIONS AND WORK CONDITIONS IN THE MERCURY MINE

Incidence of Mercury Intoxications

In the first 20 years following the second world war, the number of intoxicated miners and smelters was very high. The number of intoxicated workers represented 10 to 14% of all workers employed in the Mine. 139 and 145 cases of intoxication with mercury occurred in 1952 and 1953, respectively. In subsequent periods the number of intoxications among workers exposed to mercury decreased slightly. The relative number of intoxicated workers was during the years always higher in the smelting plant than in the mine. The index of intoxication frequency (number of intoxications per 100 workers) in the mine and in the smelting plant reached in the year 1964 practically the same value: 11 intoxications per 100 workers. In 1962 the number of intoxications among workers exposed to mercury repeatedly increased to 96 cases (Hribernik 1950, Kobal 1965) (Fig.1.).

In 1964, 104 cases of intoxication were reported; 83 were reported in 1968, 35 in 1972, and only two cases of intoxication were reported in 1975. After 1975, there were no new cases of intoxication (Fig. 2), in spite of the fact that excavation activities were moved to areas where native mercury was present (Kobal 1991).

In the period from 1960 to 1964 intoxications appeared in predominantly subacute forms in 65% of the cases, and chronic forms of intoxication appeared in 35% of the patients. There were no acute intoxications. Prevailing in the clinical picture of subacute intoxications were tremor, stomatitis, ptyalism (excessive production of saliva) and disorders of the digestive tract. In chronic cases the characteristic tremor was accompanied by "erethismus mercurialis". The clinical picture of intoxications depended primarily on the level, duration and frequency of workers' exposure to mercury vapours. Subacute forms of intoxication usually appeared after shorter periods of exposure (after 5 - 14 days) to increased concentrations of elemental mercury in air (between 0.5 - 1.0 mg/m^3). In these forms of mercury intoxications the urine mercury concentrations were very high, usually over 600 μg/L (Kobal 1975a, 1991, 1994).

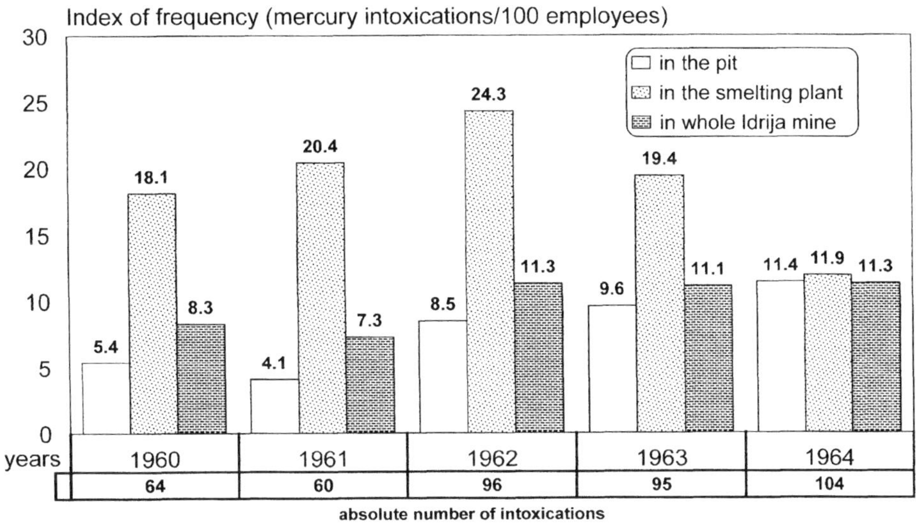

Fig 1. Incidence of occupational mercury intoxications in the Idrija Mercury Mine from 1960 to 1964

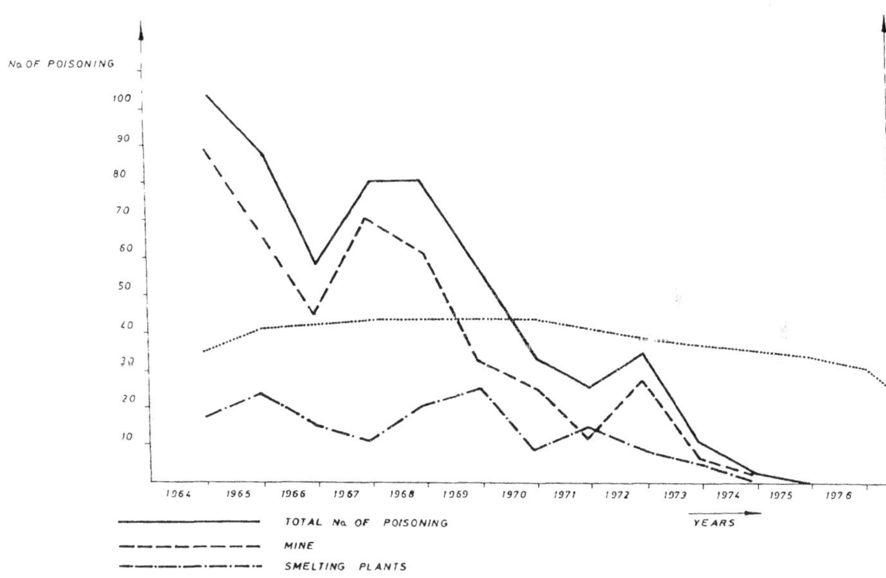

Fig 2. Mercury poisoning 1964 -1976 in the Idrija Mine

Work Conditions

The extraction of ore in the pit is predominantly a mechanized process, but partly it is also carried out manually. The dynamic loads of miners ranged on average from 5 to 9 Kcal/min., while the pulmonary ventilation during work was from 24 to 33 l of air/min (Sušnik et al. 1974, Kobal 1991). The static muscle loads were most pronounced during carpentry works. The air temperature and relative humidity in the pit mostly ranged from 15 to 27°C and from 70 to 80%, respectively. On some levels the temperature even reached 30°C and the relative humidity was as high as 92%. The air velocity ranged from 0.20 to 0.70 m/sec. Effective temperatures even reached values as high as 27.8°C. The dust level in work areas was highest during mechanical loading and discharging of ore. Particularly high values were recorded during dry drilling and blasting and during pneumatic backfilling. Before 1961 the dust level in working areas attained values of 30 to 70 mg/m^3 of air, while in the period from 1972 to 1978 the values of dust in air reached 40 mg/m^3. The share of free silica in dust primarily depended on its content in ore. The free silica content in mineralized skonca shale ranged from 10 to 35%. Increased concentrations of radon and its short-lived offspring were also found in some workplaces in the pit and skonca shales. The gamma dose-rate in mine galleries in Carboniferous shale ranged from 0.15-0.20 μGy/h, and in bituminous shale up to 1 μGy/h. Radon concentrations in upper parts of the mine were found to be 814-2122 Bq/m^3, with a peak value of 4144 Bq/m^3 in the period 1961-1970 and 700-1100 Bq/m^3, with a peak value of 1500 Bq/m^3 in the period 1991 - 1995.

In the smelting plant the concentrations of elemental mercury (Hg^0) were from 0.00 to 3.00 mg/m^3 of air. In sulphide ore excavation areas, the concentration of mercury vapours in air was predominantly below the maximum allowable concentration (MAC, 0.10 mg/m^3). In pit areas where native mercury was mined, the concentration in working and unventilated areas was very high and periodically exceeded 2.5 mg/m^3 of air and most of the time exceeded the maximum allowable levels of mercury vapours in air (0.1 mg/m^3).

Mercury appears in the air of excavation areas of the Idrija Mine in the form of vapours, aerosols and dust particles. Vapours represent over 97% of the total amount of mercury in the pit air (Valič et al. 1965, Kavčič et al. 1974).

During the period from 1952 to 1964 the main safety measures introduced at workplaces with increased mercury concentrations were: reduction of working hours (6 hours/day) and rotations of workers. The assignment of workers to workplaces with increased mercury concentrations either in the pit or the smeltery was conducted by the Technical Service, most often without any reliable data on mercury concentrations in working areas and without giving consideration to earlier exposures of workers. In this period (1952 - 1964) the technical preventive measures introduced at workplaces with elevated mercury concentrations were very deficient. The miners working in the pit did not use personal safety equipment. Only when specific tasks were performed in the smeltery did workers periodically use half-masks with anti-mercury vapour filters (Topolnik et al. 1952). The Health Service did not participate in the assignment of workers to workplaces with elevated mercury concentrations, nor did it carry out the medical surveillance of workers during regular occupational exposure, except during annual cleaning of the smeltery. Once a year the consequences of previous exposures to mercury were only determined by the mine physician during preventive medical examinations of workers.

THE HEALTH SAFETY PROGRAMME FOR WORKERS EXPOSED TO ELEMENTAL MERCURY AT THE MERCURY MINE IN IDRIJA

The work conditions in the mine urgently called for more effective preventive measures for workers' protection against exposure to mercury. A professional team was formed within the Mine, comprising experts from the Health Service, the Safety at Work Service and the chemical laboratory and technical staff. A team approach enabled the preparation of a complex health prevention programme for workers exposed to elemental mercury. The programme included technical measures for the reduction of mercury concentrations in working areas, the use of personal safety equipment, specific medical supervision and limited work load in the case of workers exposed to elevated mercury concentrations. The chemical laboratory became gradually more involved in the analysis of mercury levels in the environment and biological materials. This enabled the Health Service to intensify its activities related to the preventive health care of workers exposed to mercury.

Due to the specific type of exposure of workers to mercury in the pit, our research activities in health safety had to be directed to the validation of known indicators of the degree of exposure (WHO 1976; Roels et al. 1985, 1987). After 1985 our studies were devoted to: the relation between external exposure and the internal dose received during exposure, the kinetics of mercury elimination from the blood, the relation between blood and urine mercury during regular exposure, and catalase enzyme activity in erythrocytes during elevated mercury absorption. The results of our studies enabled us to estimate the health-based biological limit value of mercury in urine, which were used in estimating internal doses of mercury during intermittent type of exposure (Kobal 1991).

The complete health and safety program contains the following:

- regular monitoring of Hg^0 concentrations at workplaces in the pit and smelting plant,
- improvement of technical measures for the reduction of mercury concentrations at workplaces in areas with native mercury,
- continuous use of personal safety equipment by workers exposed to mercury,
- regular monitoring of external exposure of individual workers and estimation of cumulative monthly external exposure,
- regular and controlled rotation of workers from hazardous to nonhazardous workplaces and the reduction of their exposure to mercury from 6 to 4 hours daily,
- medical surveillance and estimation of workers' specific ability for work at workplaces with increased concentrations of Hg vapours.

Air Monitoring and Mercury Emission Controls

The measurement of mercury vapours is performed daily with so-called instant reading methods in all work areas with native mercury and at other important points in the pit and the smelting plant. They are generally performed during every critical work phase in which the highest mercury concentrations are expected.

Test measurements of mercury vapours in the pit atmosphere and the smelting plant of the Idrija Mercury Mine began in 1956 (portable instrument). Initially, the measurements were carried out only a few times per year (19 measurements in 1956), later they were performed a few times per month (41 measurements in 1960), and since 1977 measurements of Hg vapours in the working atmosphere have been performed every work day.

Daily measurements of Hg° concentrations in the air of working areas were performed with a Beckmann Vapour Meter K-23 USA (until 1989). At present these measurements are performed with a Mercury Vapour Indicator Shawcity, UK (since 1989). Once monthly the mine laboratory performed analyses of mercury in pit air using continuous samples ($KMnO_4$) for the purpose of controlling regular minute measurements with UV indicators. The measurements of mercury concentrations in work areas were performed by a special team under the supervision of the Safety at Work service. Data on measurements at individual workplaces and the exposure times of individual workers were also used to elevate the intensity of external exposure of individual workers.

Technical Measures for the Reduction of Hg^0 in the Working Environment

The technical measures for the reduction of Hg^0 in work areas include: adequate ventilation, improvements in ore-extracting technology and the use of a calcium polysulphide CaS_n solution for watering the free surfaces in native mercury ore extraction areas aimed at preventing the vaporization of Hg^0.

Ventilation

This technical measure includes efficient front area ventilation, and, as a side effect the reduction of air temperature in the pit. Our studies were aimed at estimating the optimal flow and velocity of air to be supplied to front areas in order to prevent the accumulation of mercury vapours at workplaces. It has been proven by studies that the delivery of fresh uncontaminated air to excavation areas is beneficial. Fresh air is supplied by a separate ventilation system at a rate of 300 - 400 m^3/min (the temperature of the input air should be as low as possible) for an area of approximately 10 m^2. Forced ventilation should not raise dust (v_{max}) and the distance between the front area and the ventilation pipe should not exceed four times the length of the front ($l = 4\sqrt{F}$). The contaminated air must be led out of the excavation area through separate outlets in order to prevent the contamination of other work areas (Teply 1974).

The results of studies presented in this section indicate that it is not possible to reduce mercury vapour concentration below 0.1 mg/m^3, since its concentration at an air flow rate of 400 m^3 /min is 0.2 mg/m^3. By delivering fresh air into front areas as directly as possible, the temperature in the work area can also be reduced and with it the concentration of mercury vapours in pit air.

Calcium polysulphide solution (CaS_n)

The results of ventilation have led to the use of moisture and chemical agents to prevent the raising of dust and the formation of aerosols by air turbulence, and to achieve the coating of mercury drops. Several agents have been tested in the laboratory and in situ investigations (water, a mixture of clay and $CaCl_2$ solution, calcium polysulphide solution). The calcium polysulphide solution proved to be the most effective (Kavčič 1975). A HgS film is formed as a result of the following chemical reaction $Hg + CaS_n \rightarrow HgS + CaS_{(n-1)}$. It coats the Hg drops and prevents their evaporation. The film is very stable. The rate of the chemical reaction between the polysulphide and native Hg is increased further by mixing it with the excavated ore (Fig. 3). It follows from the above-mentioned studies that the use of calcium polysulphide solution is very effective in reducing Hg concentrations, i.e. by a minimum of 50%. This solution is stable in time and most effective if mixed with excavated ore. It is convenient for handling (for preparation of the concentrate - mix 100 g of lime and 100 g of sulphur in 1 l of water and boil for 30 minutes; dilute to a ratio of 1:10), does not pollute the air in the room and is relatively cheap, and prevents the raising of dust and the formation of aerosols.

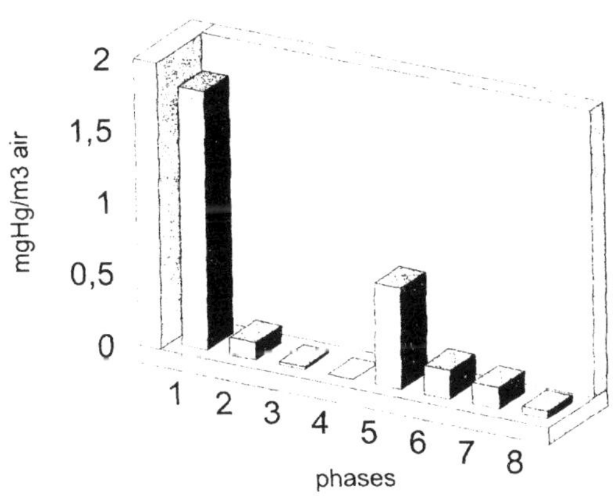

Phases of treatment:
1. before mixing
2. immediately after mixing
3. mixed, wet material
4. mixed, damp material
5. mixed, dry material
6. 30.min after mix.of dry mat.
7. 60.min after mix.of dry mat.
8. 2 days after mix.of dry mat.

Fig 3. Changes in concentrations of Hg vapours during mixing of mercury ore treated with Cas_n solution

Ore processing technology

The excavation of mineralised permocarboniferous schist containing native mercury was intensified by the development of a new underhand mining method with cemented backfill. The reduction of the active vaporization surface (surface with drops of native mercury) reduces the emission of vaporized mercury, which essentially contributes to the reduction of mercury concentrations in pit air (Bajželj 1990). From the aspect of safety at work, the main advantage of this technologically most demanding excavation method ever tested and introduced in the Idrija Mine was the reduction of the active mercury evaporation surface by 30%.

Personal safety equipment

Only after 1952 did the workers in the smeltery begin to use masks with anti-mercury vapour filters. During particularly hazardous works, e.g. during annual cleaning of the smeltery, insulating devices were used, which where later followed by the so-called "pipe half-masks" with compressed-air supply. The mask with the anti-mercury vapour filter used in the smeltery (Topolnik et al, 1952) was not suitable for work in the pit, primarily due to the high breathing resistance and the weight of the filter. In the period after 1965 the use of a half-mask with an anti-mercury vapour filter was prescribed at all workplaces in the pit where mercury concentrations in air exceeded 0.1 mg/m^3 (MAC value). Dräger's half-mask with M- 105 St filter was mostly used at the time (Fig. 4). During more strenuous physical loads in the pit, the workers could hardly use the half-mask with anti-mercury vapour filter due to the enormous effort required in respiration, as the pulmonary ventilation rose to 33 l of air per minute during the most difficult physical works. At such loads the workers rejected the use of specific safety equipment (Kobal, 1975b).

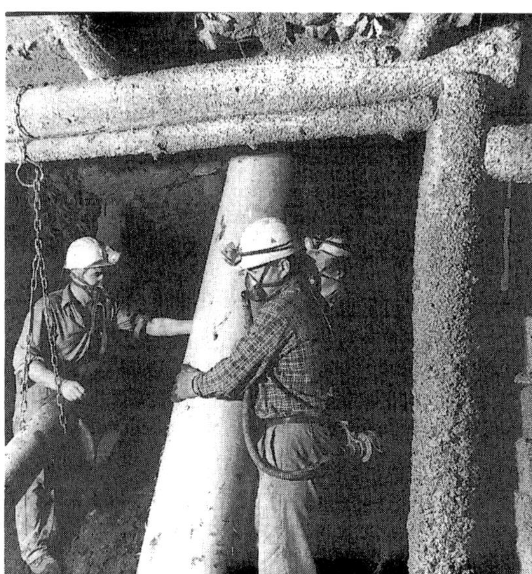

Fig 4. Miners at specific works in the pit

The English company Racal Safety Ltd., released its new protective helmet, Airstream AH, which enables the breathing of purified air through a filter. A fan installed in front of the filter is used to overcome the resistance of the filter to air flow, providing a greater supply of purified air to the miner. The AH helmet is combined with two filters, i.e. with an outer filter for coarse dust particles and a fine filter coated with two layers of activated carbon (AS 60502) for the adsorption of mercury vapours. These helmets have been widely used in dangerous work areas within the pit since 1987. During the trial phase of the use of the AH-6 helmet in the pit, the capacity of the filter was regularly controlled by continuous measurements of concentrations of elemental mercury in the air outside and inside the helmet. At a full capacity of the filter, the absorption was very good in the majority of body positions during work. The cumulative load to the two-layer activated carbon AS 60502 filter is given by $B_{max} = c \cdot t_F < 1200$ (B= filter load; c= Hg vapour concentration in the workplace, mg/m^3; t_F=duration of filter's i.e. miner's exposure to specific Hg concentrations) (Stegnar, Zvonarič, Nanut 1986). The filter in the helmet needs to be replaced after the cumulative load of $B_{max} = 1200$ points is achieved.

In the period of the protective helmet's (AH-6) introduction into pit practice, the workers (volunteers) were subjected to in-depth medical surveillance with biological monitoring (determination of Hg content in blood), which proved its effectiveness and thus justified the use of the AH-6 helmet with filter AS 60502 (Kobal 1991).

Estimation of the intensity of external monthly exposure

Since the concentrations of native mercury in the carboniferous schist excavation areas were within the range of 0.11 to 1.00 mg Hg/m^3, the daily exposure of miners was shortened to four hours. However, all miners in these areas also used AH-6 helmets. The workers' monthly cumulative external exposure, i.e. Monthly Exposure Intensity (I_M), was regularly calculated on the basis of actual concentrations and the duration of daily exposure. A starting point for the determination of Allowable I_M (AI_M) was the analysis of the duration of exposure of miners who became intoxicated with mercury in the period before the use of personal safety equipment (Kobal 1975c) and the premise that in areas where the concentration of mercury vapours attained 0.1 mg/m^3 in air (MAC value), miners could work without safety equipment for eight hours daily on average 26 days per month: AI_M = 0.1 mgHg/m3 . 8 h . 26 days/month = 20,8. The AI_M is therefore 20.8 points and while working in dangerous areas, miners were not allowed to exceed this limit. In practice, the Technical Service of the Mine calculated the monthly allowable exposure in the following manner:

$$I_M = \Sigma\, c_n \cdot t_M$$

c_n ..... daily concentration of Hg vapours
t_M..... duration of miner's exposure to a specific Hg concentration

The records on the monitoring of daily and monthly external exposure of miners (I_M), the amount of mercury excreted in the urine of miners and the opinion of the Mine's physician were and still are kept in special miners' files (documentation). These files are used by the Mine's physician in order to determine the intensity of exposure of individual miners and adopt appropriate measures. This documentation allows the Technical Service of the Mine to regularly schedule the external exposure of workers at workplaces and take immediate measures or discontinue their exposure after they have attained the AI_M. In such cases it was necessary to consult the occupational physician.

Periodic rotation of workplaces and the reduction of daily exposure to mercury

In the 18th century Scopoli (1771) recommended a six-hour work day and the rotation of miners from hazardous workplaces to less harmful ones. These are the most successful measures for avoiding the intoxication of miners with mercury. It was the rotation of miners from dangerous workplaces (in the smelting plant) to less harmful sites (the pit - cinnabar excavation areas) that remained the main protective measure against the intoxication of miners with mercury vapours for many years after the second world war. Workplaces at which the concentration of mercury vapours was too high (over 1.0 mg/m^3) were closed, work was stopped and attempts were made to improve these areas by installing ventilation. The standard in force allowed 8 hours of work per day at mercury concentrations of up to 0.1 mg Hg/m^3. At hazardous workplaces, where this concentration exceeded 0.1 mg Hg/m^3, miners worked for 6 hours a day for about one month. Where the concentrations of Hg^0 in the pit were higher (over 0.5 mg/m^3), workers' exposure was shortened to one week. After this period, miners were transferred to the uncontaminated or less contaminated workplaces (up to the 1.0 mg/m^3). The duration of exposure and the rotation of workers were controlled only by technical supervisors in the period from 1945 till 1964.

After 1975, when the excavation of native mercury in carboniferous schist with more modern excavation technology began, the working time at these workplaces was reduced, i.e. to four hours per shift per day, 5 days per week, 4 to 5 weeks continuously, depending on AI_M and on occupational physician's decision based on the medical examination and internal dose of workers' evaluation. The miners were rotated from workplaces with native mercury to noncontaminated workplaces in the pit, as well as from the smelting plant (during annual refit) into the pit and vice versa. In this way the rotation was under the direct control of the occupational physician (Kobal 1975b, Dizdarevič 1988).

MEDICAL SURVEILLANCE OF WORKERS EXPOSED TO ELEMENTAL MERCURY (HG^0)

In the period after 1965, target medical examinations and biological monitoring of individual workers were performed prior to their assignment to work at workplaces with elevated mercury concentrations, during exposure and after exposure. During exposure the examination was focused on the detection of early nonspecific symptoms and signs of mercurialism ("mercurialismus").

During examinations the existing I_M and mercury content in urine were evaluated. Urine samples taken immediately after work were used for the evaluation of current exposure.

After 1985, when mercury extraction was reoriented exclusively to the excavation of native mercury ore, the analysis of mercury content in blood was also used in the estimation of current exposure. According to experiences gained (Kobal 1991), mercury content in blood is a valid and reliable indicator of individual current exposure or the immediate post-exposure dose, while mercury content in urine (during and after exposure) is reliable predominantly on a group level (Piotrowski et al. 1975, Nakaaki et al. 1975, WHO 1976). The analysis of mercury content in blood enabled us to quickly solve certain issues related to the problem of whether increased excretion in urine during current exposure in the consequence of mercury accumulation due to previous exposure or current exposure, or for both reasons. With respect to the appearance of symptoms and signs at increased absorption of Hg^0, we decided (Kobal 1991) to use 35 μg/L (WHO 1976) as the limit value of mercury in blood. Taking into account the individual variability of mercury excretion in urine, the upper limit for the biological value of Hg in urine (95% level of reliability) was determined as 135 μg/L (U-Hg prediction based on B-Hg value 35 μg/L, $y_{U\text{-}Hg} = 1.35\ x + 14.3$, $r = 0.68$, $P = 0.000$, standard error of predictions $s_y = \pm\ 37.7$ μg/L). This biological value was used at intermittent type of exposure to Hg^0 - 4 hours per day, for our workers, at average pulomonal ventilation 27 L/min (Kobal 1991).

Immediately after completing the target examination, the Mine physician presented his opinion *on work ability*. If the limit values of mercury in the biological material were exceeded or if nonspecific symptoms and signs of micromercurialism appeared, the worker's further exposure to mercury was stopped. In such cases the workers was usually still able to perform other jobs in areas without Hg^0 loads. The temporary interruption of exposure and transfer to another job position, which occurred as a result of increased mercury absorption, usually lasted 1 to 2 months. Upon the reassignment of workers to jobs in areas with elevated mercury concentrations, the cumulative internal dose of Hg and the half-time of mercury excretion through urine as well as the results of target medical examination were taken into account.

During the medical surveillance of workers exposed to elevated concentrations of Hg^0 in the excavation of native mercury ore after 1975, no specific symptoms or signs (WHO 1976) of occupational poisoning with mercury were found, but merely a state of increased absorption. Characteristic of this state is the appearance of some nonspecific symptoms and signs of micromercurialism ("micromercurialism") (Trachtenberg 1972, WHO 1976, Kobal 1975a, 1991), accompanied by elevated mercury content in urine. The mercury concentrations in urine most frequently ranged from 60 - 150 μg/L. In some cases without nonspecific symptoms and signs of "micromercurialism", the urine mercury concentrations reached the value 300 μg/L. This state of increased absorption was found in 40% of exposed workers as early as in 1974 (Kobal, Jamšek 1980), and again later on (1984 - 1987) in the excavation of native mercury ore (Fig. 5.).

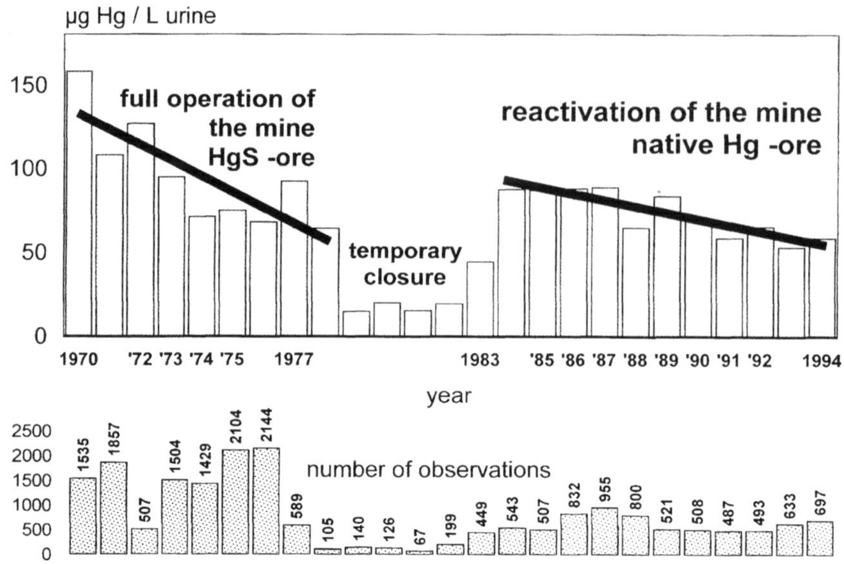

Fig 5. Mean mercury levels in the urine of exposed workers during operation of the Idrija Mercury Mine

4. Conclusion

The Health and Safety Programme for workers exposed to elemental mercury at the Idrija Mercury Mine became more extensive each year, and covered all work areas in which native mercury was mined. The implementation of the programme actually enabled a team approach to safety at work and the health safety of workers, as well as oriented applied research activities. The results of the Health and Safety Programme were very favourable; the number of mercury-intoxicated workers dropped. In spite of the fact that the excavation of native mercury was intensified in the years after reactivation of the mercury mine, the internal doses of urine mercury on a group level (in the period 1984 - 1989) did not exceed the critical level of biological limit value. In fact, the biological monitoring and medical surveillance of workers in the critical phase of exposure prevented the increased absorption and accumulation of mercury in exposed workers, and thus also the appearance of intoxication. In concluding, it should be noted that this programme was prepared for and introduced in specific underground conditions, and thus should not be generalized as a solution for the very different conditions found elsewhere.

References

Bajželj, U.: 1990, Nova odkopna metoda v zvezi s pridobivanjem živosrebrne rude v karbonskih skrilavcih s posebnim ozirom za zdravje in varnost zaposlenih, Končno poročilo, Rudarski inštitut Ljubljana.

Barber, TE., Wallis, G.: 1986, Correction of Urinary Mercury concentration by specific Gravity, Osmolality and Creatinine, Journal of Occupational Medicine, 28:354-359.

Dizdarevič, T.: 1988, Precautions for miner's protection against mercury vapours in the areas with increased mercury concentrations in the air, Graduation thesis, Univercity in Ljubljana, FNT, Slovenia in slovenian).

Hatch, WR., Ott, WL.: 1968, Determination of submicrogram quantites of mercury by atomic absorbtion spectrophotometriy, AnalytChem, 40:2085-2087.

Horvat, M.: 1989, Developement and study of analytical methods for determination of low level mercury concentration and its aplication in analysis of biological and other environmental samples, University of Ljubljana, Slovenija.

Hribernik, I.: 1950, Naša opazovanja o pofesionalnem zastrupljenju z živim srebrom v Idriji, Arhiv za higijenu rada, I:291-299.

Kavčič, I..: 1975, Raziskave vplivov fizikalnih in kemijskih parametrov na intenziteto izhlapevanja živega srebra, Separat Sigurnost u rudnicima, Zvezek 3, Beograd.

Kobal, A.: 1965, Problematika merkurializma Rudnika živega srebra v Idriji, not published (internal report).

Kobal, A.: 1975a, Professional exposure to inorganic mercury and the alterations in serum proteins, M. Sc. Thesis, University of Zagreb (in slovenian).

Kobal, A.: 1975b, Beurteilung der Wirksamkeit von persönlichen Schutzausrüstungen an Arbeitsplätzen mit hohen Konzentrationen von Quecksilberdämpfen, Zentralblatt für Arbeitsmedizin, 25:336-371.

Kobal, A.: 1975c, Ocena delovnih pogojev ekspozicije ter predlog spremembe navodila o dovoljenem času ekspozicije Hg hlapom delavcev, ki delajo na OP Karbon z dobivalnim strojem AM 50, NZD Obratna ambulanta RŽSI, Idrija, not published (internal report).

Kobal, A., Jamšek, Z.: 1980, Ocena delovne sposobnosti delavcev in varstvenih ukrepov na deloviščih s povišanimi koncentracijami anorganskega živega srebra, RŽS Idrija, not published (internal report).

Kobal, A.: 1988, Ekološka spremljava in zdravstveni nadzor delavcev na Karbonu v letu 1988, NZD Obratna ambulanta RŽSI, Idrija.

Kobal, A.: 1991, Occupational exposure to elemental mercury and its influence on mercury in blood, erythrocytes, plasma, exhaled breath and urine, and catalase activity in erythrocytes, Ph. D. Thesis, Univercity of Ljubljana, Slovenia.

Kobal, A.: 1994, Quecksilber aus Idrija - Historisch und aktuell- ein arbeitsmedizinische Betrachtung, Zbl Arbeitsmed, 44:200-210.

Mohorič, I.: 1960, Zgodovina idrijskega rudnika, Mestni muzej Idrija.

Nakaaki, K., Fukobari, S., Tada: 1975, An experimental stuy of inorganic mercury vapour exposure, J Science of Labor, 12:705-716.

Piotrowski, J., Trojanowska, B., Mozilnicka, EM.: 1975, Excretion kinetics and variability of urinary mercury in workers exposed to mercury vapour, IntArchOccupEnvironHealth, 35:245-256.

Roels H, et al.: 1985, Surveillance of workers Exposed to Mercury Vapour: Validation of a Previously Proposed Biological Thereshold Limit Value for Mrecury Concentration in Urine, American Journal of Industrial medicine 7:45-71.

Roels H, Abdeladim S, Ceulemans E, Lauwerys R.: 1987, Raelationship between the concentrations of mercury in air and in blood or urine in workers exposed to mercury vapour, Ann occup Hyg 2:135-145.

Scopoli, JA.: 1771, De Hydrargyro Idriensi Tentamina Physico-Chymico-Medica, Janae et Lepsiae (2nd edition).

Stegnar, P., Zvonarič, T., Nanut, E.: 1986, Poročilo o preizkusu učinkovitosti filtrov AS60502 proti param Hg, not published (internal report).

Sušnik, J., Kavčič, I., Verhovnik, I.: 1974, Ekološka in fiziološka analiza delovnih mest rudarjev v Rudniku živega srebra Idrija , Inštitut za medicino dela Ljubljana, Slovenija, not published (internal report).

Teply, E.: 1975, Študija eksploatacije samorodnega živega srebra v karbonskih skrilavcih Rudnika živega srebra Idrija, Rudarski inštitut Ljubljana.

Topolnik, Z., Fugaš, M., Vouk, V.B.: 1952, Zaštita radnika u Rudniku žive u Idriji, Zagreb.

Trahtenberg, IM.: 1972, The cronic action of mercury on the organism, Current aspects of the problem of micromercurialism and its prophylaxis, Kiev: ZDROV'JA 1969; summarised in: Friberg, L., Vostal, J., eds., Mercury in the environment, Chap. 7. Cleveland: The Chemical Rubber Company.

Valić, F., Morris B., Jacobs: 1965, Assesment of Mercury Air Concentrations in a Work Environment, Industrial Hygiene Journal, 266-269.

World Health Organization: 1976, Task group on Environmental Health, Environmental Health Criteria 1-Mercury, Geneva.

Zielhuis, RL.: 1978, Biological monitoring. Scand J Work Environ Health, 4:1-18.

Exposure to metallic mercury in workers in a tropical chloralkali plant evaluated through urine analysis, Rio de Janeiro, Brazil.

MALM, O; CALASANS, C.F.; FERNANDES, A. P.; BASTOS, W.R. AND PFEIFFER, W.C.

Instituto de Biofísica Carlos Chagas Filho. Universidade Federal do Rio de Janeiro (UFRJ). CCS, Ilha do Fundão, 21949-900. RJ. Brasil

Abstract: Occupational exposure to Hg vapour was investigated in 78 workers during three periods with different temperatures: August 1991, December 1991, and February 1992. Each individual was sampled twice in each period; before and after a six working days period (with a two free days interval). As an attempt to normalise Hg excretion urine was sampled always after a normal 8 hours night sleeping and immediately frozen. Mineralisation was done with acid and oxidant mixture and determination by cold vapour Atomic Absorption Spectrophotometry (Varian VGA-76 and AA-1475). Analytical accuracy was controlled by routine analysis of certified reference material (Seronorm TM trace elements, Nycome As diagnostics Olso - Norway) and all samples were analysed in triplicates. Of a total of 355 samples analysed 13% were over the maximum limit for occupational exposure (50 $\mu g.l^{-1}$ or ppb). From the 78 individuals investigated 13% presented average value smaller than 10 ppb; just 8% had the average over 50 ppb; 64% showed averages smaller than 30 ppb; and 28% were between 30 and 50 ppb. Seasonal variation was observed with the highest values in the hottest periods. High variability was observed in the same individual even within an interval of just few days (seven days). No increase of Hg in urine after the six days of exposure was observed when compared with the values after the two free days interval.

1. Introduction

Metallic Hg is liquid at room temperature and compared with other metals is highly volatile. Vapour pressure is also high and very dependent on temperature being around 14 $\mu g.m^{-3}$ at 20°C and 72 $\mu g.m^{-3}$ at 100°C (Andren e Nriagu, 1979).

Due to its very peculiar characteristic of forming amalgams with several metals, Hg is used for several purposes as well as in many industries, among them the chloralkali plants.

The basic of the process at those industries consists of an electrolytic process over a concentrated solution of NaCl where metallic Hg, (Hg^0) is used as a cathode, forming an amalgam with sodium. Afterwards the amalgams react with water producing caustic soda (NaOH) and releasing chlorine gas (Cl_2). Hg is also released and reused in the process (Nriagu, 1979), but losses occur to air, water bodies and surrounding soils.

The main purpose of this work was to evaluate the exposure of workers from a chloralkali plant situated in a hot situation in a tropical city, Rio de Janeiro, Brasil.

2. Toxicology

Mercuric ion is toxic to human beings because its affinity with sulfhydryl (S-H) groups in proteins. The combination of Hg with those groups can interfere in biological process mediated by enzymes. Hg vapour is readily absorbed by lungs, transported by blood and due to its lipossolubility accumulate in nervous cells.

Oxidation of Hg^0 to Hg^{2+}, is partially done in blood by red cells but also in other tissues after distribution. Oxidation sometimes is not fast enough to avoid Hg^0 to cross hemato-encephalic barrier. This oxidation reduces accumulation on critic organs as cerebrum and foetus (WHO, 1991). Kidneys are the main fate of inorganic (Hg^{2+}) after exposure to Hg^0. Inorganic Hg is excreted through urine and feces, with half life at urinary system between 40 and 60 days (Barregård, 1993; Sälsten Barregårg and Schütz, 1993). According to these authors the half life of Hg in blood after long term exposure to Hg vapours is 3.8 (3.1 - 5.1) days in the fast phase and 45 (28 - 121) days in the slow phase.

Early signs of Hg^0 contamination are associated with dysfunctions on the nervous system (insomnia, irritability, loss of memory) but also some locally affected areas (gingivitis). Other main symptoms are: bronchitis, headache, mercurialentis, tremor, weakness, renal failure, interstitial pneumonitis, mercurialism (with erethism), parestesia, reduction of libido and intellectual capacity (WHO, 1991). Several symptoms are not very specific so analyses on corporal fluids or tissues (when possible) are necessary.

Total Hg in urine was used as the best indicator of inorganic Hg body burden for evaluation of workers exposed to metallic Hg in a chloralkali plant.

Concentrations under 7 $\mu g\ Hg.l^{-1}$ urine can be considered normal for people not exposed and 50 $\mu g.l^{-1}$ (WHO,1991). the maximum acceptable value for occupationally exposed population, corrected to the creatinine value ($50\mu g\ .g^{-1}$.creatinine)

3. Material and Methods

Sampling was done in a systematic way, the workers collected at home their first urine in the morning in polyethylene flasks (250 ml) previously washed with HNO_3 5%. Samples were immediately frozen and transported to Instituto de Biofísica Carlos Chagas Filho - UFRJ, and analysed within a period of 48 hours.

Orientation for the workers was provided regarding care in sampling to avoid contamination. Blanks of the sampling procedure were performed by the workers also.

Occupational exposure to Hg vapour was investigated in 78 practical workers responsible for routine operation and maintenance of the industrial plant during three periods along seven months;

- **August 1991, with mild temperatures (ranging from 21 - 33 °C);**
- **December 1991, with very hot temperatures (ranging from 26 - 40 °C) and;**
- **February 1992, with very hot temperatures (ranging from 27 - 40°C).**

Each individual was sampled twice in each period: after a six working days period and after a two free days interval at home; so each worker should provide six samples.

As an attempt to normalise data on Hg excretion, urine was sampled after a normal 8 hours night sleep.

Air Hg concentrations were measured in some situations during a 2 hour period in different parts of the chloralkali plant. Sampling was done bubbling air through an acidic and oxidant solution at a flow rate of around 1 $l.min^{-1}$. Seventeen air samples were collected in the two main electrolysis plants. Unfortunately those air samples were only possible during the end of September when local temperatures should be mild but it was not. Average temperature was 32 °C with values ranging from 22 °C to 41 °C during the last 15 days of September. During summer temperature in the area can reach 45 °C.

ANALYSIS OF MERCURY

Urine: Mineralisation was done with acid mixture (HNO_3 and H_2SO_4), heated to 60°C, followed by oxidant solution of $KMnO_4$ 5 %, heated again and then an overnight pause. Next day excess oxidants were reduced with some drops of NH_4ClO 12% and determination was done by cold vapour Atomic Absorption Spectrophotometry (Varian VGA-76 and AA-1475).

Analytical accuracy and precision were controlled by routine analysis of certified reference material (Seronorm TM trace elements, Nycome As diagnostics Olso - Norway) and all samples were analysed in triplicates.

Air: In bubbling solution excess oxidants were reduced with some drops of NH_4ClO 12% and determination was done by cold vapour Atomic Absorption Spectrophotometry (Varian VGA-76 and AA-1475).

OTHER PARAMETERS:

An occupational as well as alimentary survey was performed, aiming to detect any other possible Hg source, including number of amalgams, fish-eating habits.

An interview performed by a medical doctor student (author) and the first author looking for symptoms and signs (clinical examination) of Hg intoxication were also performed with 89 workers with half to 28 years working in the industry (average: 10.6 years; standard deviation: 7.9; median: 10 years) aiming at identification of more general evident health disturbances. Symptoms like micturarion disturbances, reduction of visual acuity, loss of hearing, sialorrhea, violent muscular spasms, diarrhoea, abdominal pain, stomatitis, polydipsia, dyspnoea, fatigue, insomnia and loss of memory were inquired to the workers. Signs like, rest tremor, teeth loosening, and dermatitis, were searched through clinical examination. History of pneumonia and gout were also inquired.

Some biochemical parameters of urine samples as density, leukocytes, nitrite, protein, pH, glucose, cetonic corps, uroblinogen and bilirubin were determined through strip paper test (Combur 10 Test^R), as extra information on general clinical situation of individuals as well as for checking authenticity and/or abnormalities in the samples.

4. Results and Discussion

Minoia *et al.* (1990), after determining the Hg concentrations in urine in 380 healthy individuals not exposed to Hg obtained an average concentration of 3,5 ± 0,2 $\mu g.l^{-1}$ and established reference values for non-exposed populations ranging from 0,1 a 6,9 $\mu g.l^{-1}$. According to those authors the threshold values for first metabolic changes is around 16,5 $\mu g.l^{-1}$. Control individuals at our institute without any direct exposure presented values always smaller than 8 ppb.

Air Hg concentrations (N = 17) ranged from 1 $\mu g.m^{-3}$ to 64 $\mu g.m^{-3}$ inside the electrolysis areas with an average value around 25.5 $\mu g.m^{-3}$. Just three samples were above the maximum limit for occupational exposure (50$\mu g.m^{-3}$) established by the WHO(1991).

Summary of the data regarding the average value of individuals: (see also Figure 1)

- The 78 workers evaluated over the 3 periods showed a final average value around 27 $\mu g.l^{-1}$ urine.
- 13% of the them presented average value smaller than 10 $\mu g.l^{-1}$;
- 64% showed average smaller than 30 $\mu g.l^{-1}$ and;
- Just 8% of them had the average over 50 $\mu g.l^{-1}$ (acceptable limits for workers occupationally exposed to Hg);
- 28% were between 30 and 50$\mu g.l^{-1}$.

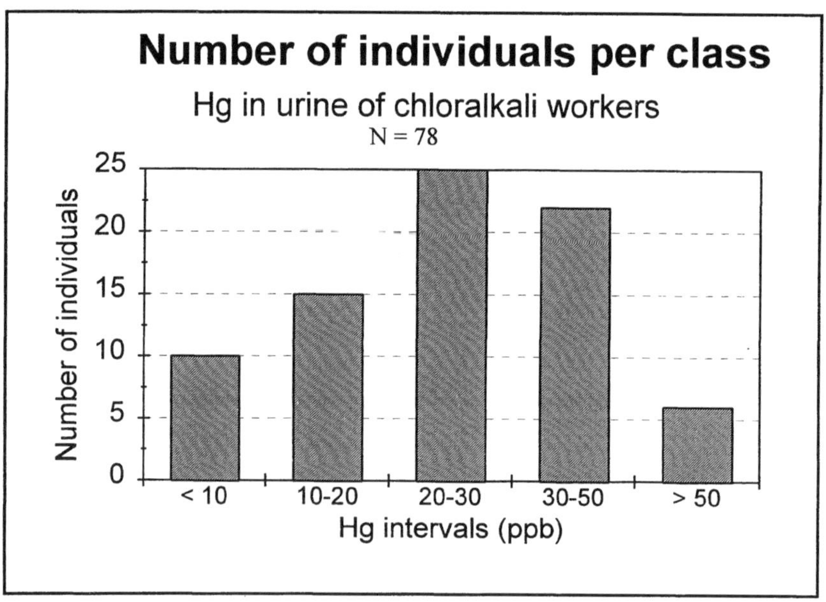

Figure 1.

If we consider the total number of samples collected as one group of data a very similar figure (see Figure 2) is obtained with the distribution of data a deviated to a a lower level class, of Hg concentrations value indicating that high variability for the in some individuals, reducing the average distribution when considering all samples together.

Summary of the data obtained regarding all the urine samples together:

- Of a total of 355 samples analysed 12% were over the maximum permissible concentration for occupational exposure (50 $\mu g.l^{-1}$);
- 18% were smaller than 10 $\mu g.l^{-1}$;
- 65% were smaller than 30 $\mu g.l^{-1}$.

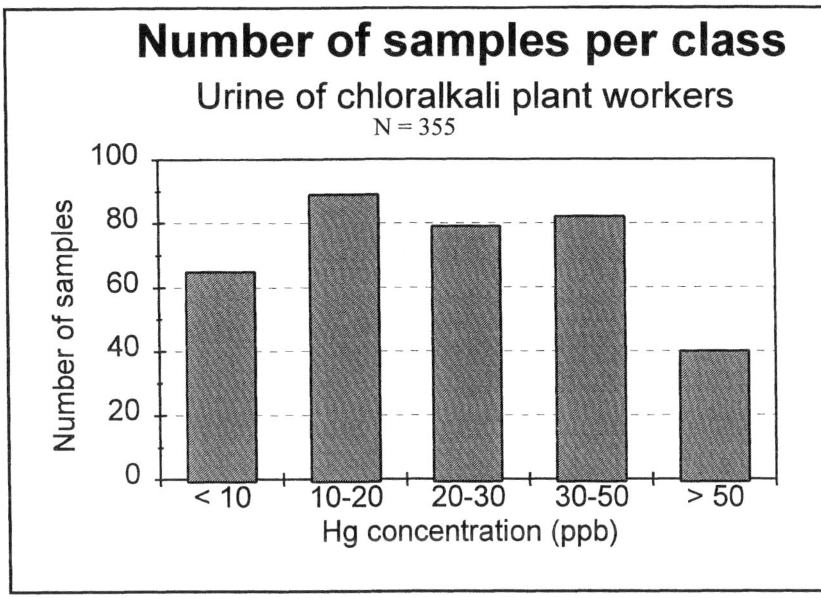

Figure 2.

Seasonal variation was observed with the highest urine values in the hottest periods. (See Table 1).

Table 1: Seasonal variation of Average, Minimum, and Maximum concentrations of Hg ($\mu g.l^{-1}$) and coefficient of variation (%) in urine of workers from a chloralkali plant.

Month	Average	Minimum	Maximum	C.V.
August (with mild temperatures)	23.6	1.5	64.1	61
December (very hot temperatures)	33.0	0.8	136.7	74
February (very hot temperatures)	25.4	0.9	119.4	83

No trend of increasing Hg in urine after the six days of exposure was observed when compared with the values after the two free days interval at home. This is probably related with the high half life of Hg in urine.

Variability on Hg levels between workers was higher during hottest periods as can be seen in table 1.

High variability on Hg levels was observed in the same individual. In some cases individuals with average values higher than 30 $\mu g.l^{-1}$ also presented values close to normality just sampling 3 days after.

As an illustration of this variability some examples of representative individuals, with coefficient of variation of six samples as well as maximum and minimum values of the same person within 3 days are presented in Table 2.

Table 2: Coefficient of Variation, Average and minimum and maximum Concentrations of Hg ($\mu g.l^{-1}$) in urine (with 3 days interval with no exposure) of workers from a chloralkali plant. Representative cases.

Individual	Coefficient of Variation % (N=6)	Average (N=6)	Minimum and Maximum from a 72 hours interval (N=2)	
X	10.25	32.7	31.6	32.3
Y	45.4	27.8	5.1	28.8
K	47.4	47.4	55.4	106.1
Z	75.7	28.2	23.3	69.4

Several complaints were observed after clinical examination and interview with the workers.

The frequency (in percentage of individuals with positive response) of most common symptoms or signs based on affirmation of the workers (interview) or through medical examination were:

- Memory disturbances 69 %
- Reduction of visual acuity 40 %
- Insomnia 35 %
- Fatigue 32 %
- Micturation disturbances 30 %
- Polidypsia 26 %
- Dyspnoea 21 %
- Violent muscular spasm 22 %
- Sialorrhea 19 %
- Dark urine in the morning 15 %

When only individuals that presented levels higher than 50 $\mu g.l^{-1}$ are considered the main complaint was reduction of visual acuity but with similar frequency with individuals with urine Hg between 30 and 50 ppb. Average frequency of complaints was 22% higher in the group with 30 - 50 ppb than in the individuals with urine Hg > 50 ppb. Just three of the symptoms and signs were higher in the group with more than 50 ppb: dermatitis, fatigue and sialorrhea. No direct relation between the gravity of complaints and Hg concentrations was observed. Frequency of complaints in individuals with Hg urine values higher than 50 ppb were lower than in the ones with concentrations ranging from 30 to 50 ppb.

5. Conclusions

Most of the individuals obtained Hg urine averages 2 to 5 times higher than the limit for non-exposed populations (WHO, 1991).

Nevertheless 92% of the workers had average values under maximum permissible concentration for occupational exposure (50 $\mu g.l^{-1}$).

Despite the fact that 76% of individuals investigated presented levels higher than the limit that triggers metabolic changes (16,5 $\mu g.l^{-1}$), no relation was observed between clinical examination and Hg concentrations.

Acknowledgements: Financial support: CNPq, Pan-Americana SA

References

Andren, A.W. e Nriagu, J.O. 1979. The global cycle of mercury. In: The biogeochemistry of mercury in the environment. Nriagu, J.O. (Ed.) Amsterdam: Elsevier/ North Holland Biomedical Press,. 696 p. p. 1-15.

Barregård, L. 1993. Biological monitoring of exposure to mercury vapour. Scand. J. Work Environ. Health. 19 suppl 1:45-9.

World Health Organization (WHO). 1991. Environmental Health Criteria, 118. Inorganic Mercury -. Geneva, 168 p.

Sällsten, G., Barregård, L and Schütz, A. 1993. Decrease in mercury concentration in blood after long term exposure: a kinetic study of chloralkali workers. British Journal of Industrial Medicine. 50: 814-821.

Minoia, C., Sabbioni, E., Apostoli, P. *et al.* 1990. Trace element reference values in tissues from inhabitants of the european community. I. A study of 46 elements in urine, blood and serum of italian subjects. The Science of the Total Environment, v. 95, p. 89-105,

Nriagu, J. O. (Ed.). 1979. Production and uses of mercury. In: The biogeochemistry of mercury in the environment. Amsterdam: Elsevier/ North Holland Biomedical Press, 696 p. p. 23-39.

Mercury Values in Urine from Inhabitants of St. Petersburg

S. E. Pogarev [1], V. V. Ryzhov [1], N. R. Mashyanov [1] and M. B. Sobolev [2]
[1] Institute of the Earth Crust, St. Petersburg State University, 199034 St. Petersburg Russia
[2] St. Petersburg Academy of Pediatrics, 194100 St. Petersburg Russia

Abstract. The results of 3000 urine analyses are presented. The observational data were obtained for the reference group of school children and adults and for groups of people suffered from indoor mercury pollution. A novel Zeeman atomic absorption spectrometer and cold vapour and piroliz methods were used for determination of total mercury. A background mercury value in urine for St. Petersburg region is determined as 0.5 μg/l. Distributions of mercury concentrations in urine after five accidents are given. There are considerable differences in total mercury distribution for each group, that depend on level of Hg exposure. Peculiar features of the 24-hour rhythm of mercury excretion with urine is used for the treatment of patients, an optimal therapy selection and rehabilitation control.

1. INTRODUCTION

There is a number of different sources of outdoor and indoor mercury (Hg) pollution in St. Petersburg. The local haloes in ambient air, up to 150-300 ng/m^3 and more have been recorded around the city plants that use this metal in technological processes (production of electrical and control instruments, batteries, medicines), and over some dump sites (Dreval *et al*, 1996 and Mashyanov and Reshetov, 1995). Metal mercury-containing control and electrical instruments, vacuum equipment, fluorescent lamps are widespread in research and medical centres, plants and their industrial laboratories, power stations. Mercury containing thermometers are still used by people, as well as in hospitals, schools and kindergartens. Considerable amount of stored mercury (approximately 6-12 ton) is still kept at enterprises and laboratories of the city, at least 3-3.5 ton — at flats, in home thermometers and tonometers. As a rule, it is a regular source of accidents connected with spilling of metal mercury on the city territory and inside buildings. Annually, municipal emergency service records 200-250 accidents of indoor and outdoor pollution, 10-20 of them major (of over 1 kg) resulting in damage to both industrial structures and housing (Dreval *et al*, 1996). Therefore, important is the timely selection and curing the victims of mercury vapor inhalation.

Due to the simplicity of sampling and preparation, urinalysis is the most common means of evaluating the exposure effects to people of Hg pollution in the environment and work place. In common medical practice, a total mercury content in urine of up to 10 μg/l is considered normal in Russia. Although, the additional research has shown that even though there are no explicit signs of poisoning, changes in the immune system and other adverse affects take place among workers regularly contacting with mercury, despite allowable mercury levels in urine of less than 5 μg/l (Aladatov *et al*, 1990). There is no consensus on safe mercury contents in urine. Systematic investigations dealing with mercury levels in urine for the St. Petersburg region are still lacking.

2. EXPERIMENTAL

At St. Petersburg University a portable, multipurpose atomic absorption mercury spectrometer PA-915 has been developed for mercury measurement in ambient air and any gas media, as well as in solid and liquid samples of complex composition (Sholupov and Ganeyev, 1995). The original scheme of the application of the direct Zeeman effect provides very high selective determinations. The distinguishing feature of this newly developed method is that it allows direct measurements of total Hg in environmental media without any preconcentration accumulation of mercury in a sorbent, with simultaneous controls for non-selective absorption in dynamic regimes. In order to analyse liquid and solid samples, the device has appendages working on the cold vapour and pyrolize principles to release mercury from samples. The instrument's parameters make it possible to simplify sample preparations, to detect mercury at rather low levels in samples of complex compositions, and to improve substantially the reproducibility and accuracy of analysis (Ganeyev *et al*, 1995 and Pogarev *et al*, 1995).

Strong basic stannous dichloride solution is used to destroy the mercury compounds in urine and to reduce Hg^{++} (Pogarev *et al*, 1995). The detection limit is on the range of 0.1 μg/l for the 5 ml samples. The accuracy of measurement is about 10 percent. The piroliz method has been applied to be certain that all amount of mercury is analysed. In the piroliz process all mercury compounds that may occur in the sample are bound to be broken-up by high temperature and the determination of total mercury is provided (Ganeyev *et al*, 1995). The parallel results, obtained by these two methods for urine with different mercury content, does not show an increase of the mercury exit in the piroliz case in comparison with the cold vapour method. Tested samples were taken from people breathing the air polluted by mercury vapour. We have not disposed of samples connected with mercury input by contaminated food.

3. RESULTS AND DISCUSSION

With the help of the Zeeman atomic absorption mercury spectrometer, analyses of urine samples from about 3000 persons were conducted in the manner described above.

THE BACKGROUND GROUP

The background (reference) group (380 people) was taken from valid school children and adults. Mercury content in the samples varies between less than 0.1 μg/l and 40 μg/l, although in 90 per cent of the samples mercury concentration does not exceed 2 μg/l, and in 70 per cent—0.5 μg/l. A histogram of background distribution is displayed in Figure 1. Based on this distribution we determined a background mercury value in urine for the St. Petersburg region as 0.5 μg/l. For example, this level for inhabitants of European community varies from 0.3 to 3.5 μg/l (Kramer *et al*, 1995 and Minoila *et al*, 1990).

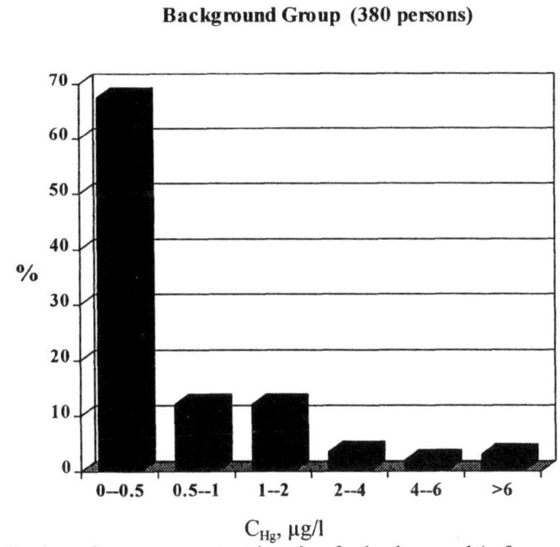

Fig. 1. Histogram of distribution of mercury content in urine for background (reference) group (380 person).

RISK GROUPS

The risk groups were comprised from dwellers of different block buildings where 0.5 - 1 kg of metallic mercury had been accidentally spilled. Urinalysis of risk groups reveals intoxicated persons (with mercury content in urine more than 1 μg/l) who need further medical treatment. The distributions of Hg concentrations in urine for five risk groups (more than 100 persons in each group) and background group are represented on the Table I.

TABLE I.

Distributions of mercury content in urine from 5 risk groups (G1-G5) and background group (G0). Number of sufferers is determined from number of person in the risk group with respect to the background group. C_{ave} - the average value Hg content in urine for suffered persons in risk group.

	Number of persons in group	Distribution of Hg concentration in urine, %				Suffered persons		
		0-1 μg/l	1-4 μg/l	4-10 μg/l	> 10 μg/l	Number	%	C_{ave} μg/l
G1	134	11.5	36	26.5	26	115	86	7.8
G2	230	16	44	24	16	184	80	6.5
G3	107	19	58	17	6	81	76	4.5
G4	101	54	33	11	2	32	32	4.3
G5	210	50	42	7	1	79	38	3.1
G0	380	80	15	3	2	--	--	--

These results were obtained in St. Petersburg during 1995. Distribution of mercury content, percent of sufferers (from 32% to 86%) and average value Hg content in urine (from 3.1μg/l to 7.8μg/l) differ considerably for each group and depend on level of Hg exposure. The statistical data permit us to compare the accident's scales using number of sufferers and the average value Hg content in urine of intoxicated persons.

DAILY MONITORING OF MERCURY EXCRETION

A successful treatment requires a most comprehensive idea about the dynamics of the toxicant being driven off the body of a patient. In this respect, we have investigated the 24-hour rhythms of mercury excretion with urine. The dynamic was investigated by collecting the urine throughout the initial screening days every 3 hours according to the conventional Zimnitsky sampling procedure.

For comparison of the changes in mercury concentration in urine samples obtained from various patients, there was used a reduced value of K_i, being the percentage ratio of the current concentration C_i and the daily maximum C_{max} ($K_i = C_i/C_{max} \times 100\%$) per patient. The Table II presents the data on the daily rate of the mercury excretion with urine (K_i) obtained for twenty children. Eligible patients were those whose reliable mercury contents in urine C_{max} exceeded 1 µg/l, unequivocally suggesting their direct contact with mercury vapours. The revealed maximum concentrations differed in the patients by almost two hundred times (patients P1, P20) which attested to the differences in dose of mercury and the individual response. All patients had their urine Hg contents significantly varying during the day; the peak concentrations exceeded the minimum values by 4-50 times (patients P2, P20). A characteristic feature of the 24-hour outflow cycle was the morning maximum (at 6-12 a.m.).

TABLE II.
Daily variance of relative mercury content in urine K_i from 20 patients (P1-P20). $K_i = C_i/C_{max} \times 100\%$, C_{max} - maximal daily value.

Patient	C_{max} µg/ l	K_i, % SAMPLING PERIOD, HOURS 0-3	3-6	6-9	9-12	12-15	15-18	18-21	21-24
P1	*1.3*	56	100	75	25	25	11	39	56
P2	*1.3*	92	100	57	77	21	70	36	25
P3	*1.7*	33	100	18	19	10	33	9	16
P4	*1.9*	26	29	100	18	50	16	16	11
P5	*1.9*	34	40	29	58	15	100	16	22
P6	*2.1*	33	100	100	90	17	14	52	43
P7	*2.1*	-	100	95	19	30	14	19	28
P8	*2.3*	30	56	100	47	24	20	14	24
P9	*2.3*	12	36	100	28	48	15	6	13
P10	*3.5*	20	14	100	16	14	22	10	8
P11	*3.5*	40	49	37	100	71	77	24	54
P12	*3.8*	16	100	21	15	16	11	11	26
P13	*4.4*	11	46	100	41	25	39	30	19
P14	*5.5*	18	27	58	100	22	20	78	78
P15	*5.6*	46	70	100	100	13	5	15	17
P16	*5.6*	100	-	-	78	98	34	18	39
P17	*6.6*	23	68	36	27	33	27	100	29
P18	*7.1*	94	65	92	100	90	40	54	51
P19	*15.*	17	-	100	32	2	-	10	7
P20	*220.*	2	2	100	3	25	28	3	2

A comparative analysis of the 24-hour cycle dynamics revealed three basic excretion types: *normal, abnormal, and permanent.* The first, normal type, is characterized by one morning peak greatly exceeding all other values (patients P8, P10, P12, P15) and resembles the standard physiological rhythm. Clinically this is revealed exclusively through vegetative dysfunction. The dynamic process of the first kind is represented in Figure 2a with histogram P10.

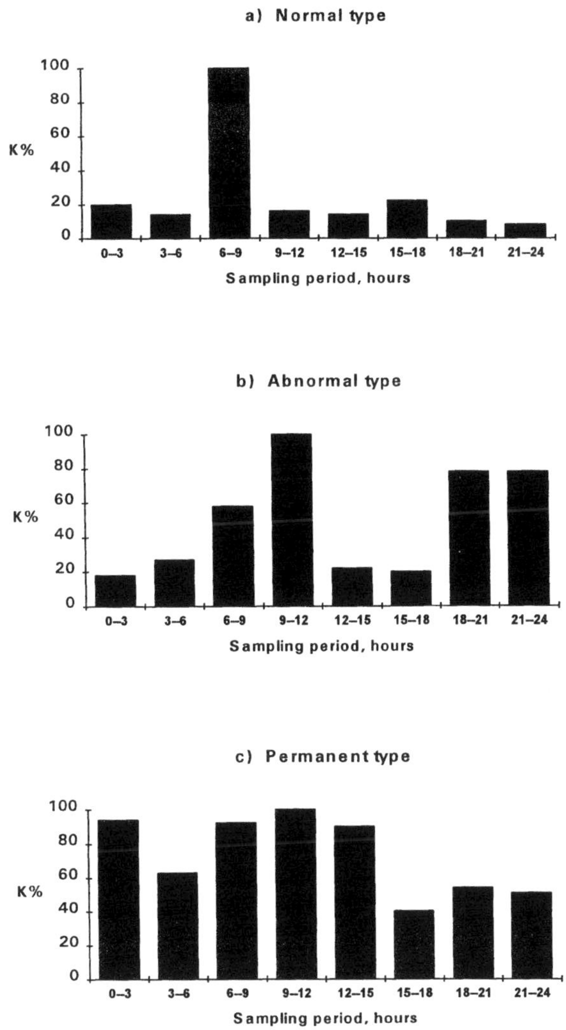

Fig. 2. Histograms of the daily variance of relative mercury content in urine. $K_i=C_i/C_{max}\times100\%$, C_{max}- maximal daily value. a) Normal type (P10, C_{max}=3.5 μg/l); b) Abnormal type (P14, C_{max}=5.5 μg/l); c) Permanent type (P18, C_{max}=7.1 μg/l).

The abnormal type has, beside the morning peak, another one occurring in the day-time or in the evening, although a much less intensive one (patients P2, P3, P4, P6, P7, P9, P14, P20). The degree to which the evening maximum is pronounced corresponds to the severity of the kidney involvement. In certain cases, it is possible to discuss a state transitional between these two types (patient P7). The abnormal type is represented on the Figure 2b with histogram P14.

The permanent type is characterized by a more uniform content of mercury in the urine with relatively insignificant variations during the day (patients P1, P5, P11, P16, P17, P18) which reflects the involvement of both the kidneys and other organs and systems. The third type is represented on the Figure 2c with histogram P18.

The analysis of the varying daily excretion cycle, the 24-hour monitoring of mercury being driven away with urine, is a way to not only reliably determine the cases of patients having direct contacts with mercury, but also to evaluate the severity of each particular case, and to predict the probability of other organs and systems being involved in the pathological process at the pre-clinical stage. The 24-hour monitoring method allows for an optimal therapy to be selected, to avoid certain consequences of careless therapy and to control the efficiency.

ACKNOWLEDGEMENTS

The authors acknowledge Institute of the Earth Crust of St. Petersburg University, Academy of Pediatrics and Rehabilitation Centre "Primorsky", which supported this research.

REFERENCES

Aladatov, A. G. Metiel, N. N. and Riebiena, G. A.: 1990, *Medikobiologicheskoye Znacheniye Urovnya Soderzhaniya Rtuti v Biosredakh Organizma*. Gigiyena i Sanitariya, **5**, pp. 88-95, (in Russian).

Dreval, T.V. Mashyanov, N.R. Ryzhov, V.V. et al.:1996, *Mercury in the Atmosphere of St. Petersburg - Distribution, Origins and Influence on Human Health.* Proc. 4th Intern. Conf. "Mercury as a Global Pollutant", Hamburg, Germany, p. 217.

Ganeyev, A A. Pogarev, S. E. Ryzhov, V. V. Sholupov, S. E. and Dreval, T. V.: 1995, *The New Method for Direct and Express Determination of Mercury in Oil, Gas Condensate and Biological Samples*. Ecol. Chem., **4**, pp. 122-126.

Kramer, D. Piechotowski, I. Jovanovik, S. et al.: 1995, *Amalgamfullungen und Quecksibergehalte im Spontanurin von Kingern Zenterable*. Hyg. und Umweltmet, **197**, pp. 296-300.

Mashyanov, N. R. and Reshetov, V.V.: 1995, *Geochemical Ecological Monitoring Using the Remote Sensing Technique*. Sci. of the Total Environ., **159**, pp. 169-175.

Minoila, C. Sabbioni, E. Apostoli, P. et al.:1990, *Trace Element Reference ValuesiIn Tissues from Inhabitants of the European Community*, Sci. of the Total Environ., **95**, pp. 89-105.

Pogarev, S. E. Ryzhov, V. V. Dreval, T. V. and Mashyanov, N. R.: 1995, *Using Zeeman Atomic Absorption Spectrometer for Mercury Detection in Urine*. Ecol. Chem., **4**, pp. 118-121.

Sholupov, S. E. and Ganeyev, A. A.: 1995, *Zeeman Absorption Spectrometry Using High Frequency Modulated Light Polarization*, Spectrochim. Acta, **50B**, pp. 1227-1236.

GPSR Compliance

The European Union's (EU) General Product Safety Regulation (GPSR) is a set of rules that requires consumer products to be safe and our obligations to ensure this.

If you have any concerns about our products, you can contact us on ProductSafety@springernature.com

In case Publisher is established outside the EU, the EU authorized representative is:

Springer Nature Customer Service Center GmbH
Europaplatz 3
69115 Heidelberg, Germany

FSC
www.fsc.org
MIX
Papier | Fördert gute Waldnutzung
FSC® C083411

Kolibri 360 GmbH
Ferdinand-Jühlke-Straße 7
99095 Erfurt, Deutschland
produktsicherheit@kolibri360.de